Linguistics, pragmatics and psychotherapy

Linguistics, Pragmatics and Psychotherapy

A guide for therapists

ELAINE CHAIKA, PhD
Providence College, Rhode Island

W

WHURR PUBLISHERS
LONDON AND PHILADELPHIA

© 2000 Whurr Publishers
First published 2000 by
Whurr Publishers Ltd
19b Compton Terrace, London N1 2UN, England and
325 Chestnut Street, Philadelphia PA 1906, USA

British Library Cataloguing in Publication Data
A catalogue record for this book is available from the British
Library.

ISBN 186156 025 7

Printed and bound in the UK by Athenaeum Press Ltd,
Gateshead, Tyne & Wear

Contents

31919

AEM4430

Preface

Why would mental health therapists want or need a book written by a scholar in linguistics? What does linguistics have to tell those engaged in the talking cure? The flip answer is, of course, 'plenty!' The serious answer fills the rest of this book.

A major advantage of close analyses of language is that it heightens one's conscious awareness of what is really going on in an interaction. One literally learns to hear more, to listen more deeply, and to make more connections. One aim of this book is to increase the therapist's sensitivity to clients' or patients' speech, thereby increasing the delicacy of the therapist's interpretations, an aim I believe to be best fulfilled by learning about linguistics.

Linguistics is the study of language, its structure, its role in cognition, and its role in shaping society. Most importantly for mental health therapists, linguistics also studies language from the point of view of how people use it to create their unique selves, to shape their lives, and to express their beliefs about the world. None of these language activities is necessarily overt. Indeed, most are covert. The most salient difference between human language and other communication systems is that human language is not isomorphic between message and meaning. That is, what is meant is not derivable by adding up the meanings of the individual words and grammatical forms employed by a speaker. Meaning is often far more than the sum of the parts of an utterance, or different from it entirely. It may even be less than the sum of its parts. This does not mean that one can assign meanings willy-nilly to an utterance. As this book will show, one derives meaning in principled ways derived from intense study of language use in experimental situations and social interactions.

Non-linguists, laypersons, so to speak, usually do not think of language as an object of formal study. They extract meaning without knowing why they think something means what they think it does. This doesn't mean that one needs a course in linguistics in order to understand people. Obviously, such a position is absurd. The point is that, in interpretation, and here one might want to invoke Freud and Jung, non-linguists have been willing to assign meanings to clients' utterances with no reference to the actual mechanisms used in producing and interpreting speech normally, so that perfectly ordinary statements have been made to take on meanings completely underivable from what was said. Indeed, such interpretations typically have not addressed the actual words and grammar used by the patient, but on impressions of what the patient might be meaning, impressions that happily fit into the psychoanalytic theories performed by the analysts. It is no accident that a good deal of psychoanalytic and psychiatric discussion of what clients' and patients' speech means is strangely devoid of actual examples of the speech actually used. Words not recorded in writing or on tape are evanescent and ephemeral, but meaning lingers, usually without the hearer's being able to recreate for others the exact words that were used to give it. Moreover, non-linguists tend to think of language holistically, as chunks which just happen to mean. They do not dissect the language itself to prove the meaning.

In truth, many linguists themselves, being first and foremost human beings, have sometimes formed their theories upon personal intuitions about language, selecting data that reinforce their theories, rather than mucking about with real data. My own theoretical underpinnings have been proofed against the hard edge of psychotic speech, the study of which I have been engaged in for over a quarter of a century. My other research area, sociolinguistics, the study of speech in social interaction, has also been a major influence on my knowledge of how people use language. My theoretical position is quite unlike that of linguists who treat language as an algorithm, as a sentence-generating mechanism. As will be evident in this book, I count myself squarely in the camps of cognitive and functional linguistics. As such, I do not discriminate a line between linguistics and pragmatics. Some linguists, however, still do, or have done, just that.

Linguists of my bent are often called pragmatists or socio-linguists. In contrast to some of the more theoretically inclined, they record and analyse actual interactions. They examine what people really say and how listeners actually interpret what has been said. This is not to say that theoreticians don't use actual language samples in creating and justifying their theories. Of course they do. However, they are frequently willing to use as examples sentences they themselves have thought up, relying upon what Noam Chomsky always called his native speaker intuition as to what constitutes the grammatical sentences of a language. From such personal language stocks, pronouncements were – and are – made about language and the mind. Some psychiatrists and other researchers into language and mental illness, especially schizophrenia, have attempted to use such theories to explain psychoses. The results have not been very happy. They certainly haven't explained psychoses or their aetiology or even what patients mean by what they say.

Although, in graduate school, I was thoroughly indoctrinated in Chomskian linguistics, I quickly found that while it certainly contains some truth, it was not in any of its incarnations sufficient for explaining actually produced language, either in speech or in writing. In contrast, then, to the schools of theoretical linguistics which originally engaged my interest, I became an early convert to pragmatic and cognitive approaches to linguistics. Therefore, the theories presented in this book are data driven, and not based upon a priori theoretical propositions. The explanations flow from close examination of interactions between therapists and clients or patients. Even the first chapter, which deals with what I consider the most viable current model of linguistics, is based upon actual widely shared language usages. The later chapters discuss applications of pragmatics to the therapeutic situation.

Dedication

To William

Chapter 1
Linguistics

Like painters, language users coordinate forms to compose a coherent emotional landscape.[1]

Introduction

This chapter gives a brief overview of current thinking about syntax and semantics, especially as they impinge upon our understanding of actual language use in therapeutic settings. It will be shown that, contrary to the beliefs engendered by some theories of linguistics, there is no sharp dividing line between syntax and semantics. It will also be suggested that the basic syntactic unit in language use is the phrase, not the sentence. By examining both the grammar used and the words, we can uncover the speaker's unstated empathies and opinions. Whereas subsequent chapters focus on speech in case histories, this one focuses on the theories underlying interpretations of speech in therapy.

Linguistics

Because they all can speak and understand, there is a great temptation for people to think that they understand how language actually works. This means that scholars feel free to make pronouncements on language data without the benefit of studying linguistics, in a way that they'd never make pronouncements about physics or biology. It is as if some researchers do not understand the role of linguistics even if they are studying something which involves language use, certainly including any study of cognition, mental illness, or mental health therapy. However, linguistics is, in and of itself, a deep and complex object of scholarly enquiry with a highly developed set of heuristics, experimental and observational techniques. Ad hoc explanations are not admissible, although they are easy to come by because of the sheer amount of language data available from anybody who speaks. As with any other science, linguists' results have to account for all the data presented, they must be replicable by other scholars, and the findings must be extendable to new data. Given the sheer volume of language data, the task is awesome, and if theories come and go, or if scholars change their minds about what was once considered absolute truth, it is only an expression of a vital science, constantly expanding its borders.

The problem of the ubiquity of linguistic data is very real. Data can be tamed, so to speak, by eliciting language in a well-constructed interview or experimental techniques, preferably those which provide a target so that the linguistic investigator can match linguistic forms with what utterances are supposed to be saying. Alternatively, linguists can constrain their data by confining them to language used in well-defined social situations. Mere impressions of the ways one thinks people talk are not acceptable. Analyses of language production of any sort must be data driven. That is, they must be based upon whatever is actually said –or written –and be consistent with the regularities within both the language structures under investigation and the context in which they were produced.

Because language data are so copious and so easily elicited, virtually any task will yield loads of it. Researchers may then give tasks and analyse the results on data which actually explain nothing. One good example is the use of word association testing with schizophrenics. This was apparently inspired by schizophrenic associational chaining (here called *glossomania*) like

> My mother's name was Bill...And coo? St. Valentine's Day is the official start of the breedin' season of the birds. All buzzards can coo. I like to see it pronounced buzzards rightly. They work hard. So do parakeets... (from Patient X)[2]

Apparently because they knew of glossomania, Chapman, Chapman and Daut[3] gave word association tests to schizophrenics to see if they used strong or weak associations to words. No matter what the results of such testing were, it makes no difference. Normal speech is not produced on the basis of word associations. The question to ask about the schizophrenic who is glossomanic is not whether or not he or she is using weak or strong associations, but why they are uttering strings of associated words at all! It is the fact of the associating itself that needs explaining, not the kind of associating. Chapman, Chapman, and Daut found that schizophrenics gave what they termed 'strong' associations to words even if the provided context called for 'weaker' ones. Even if a case could be made for the validity of finding out that schizophrenics were more likely to use strong associations, what does this tell us about schizophrenia? Perhaps subjects use strong associations because they are cognitively impaired and unusual associations do not come so easily to their minds. Or, perhaps, the patients think the test is some kind of trap so that they give a response that is not unusual in order to placate the tester. A third possibility is that the patient is so unable to concentrate on the task that he or she just gives the obvious answer to the target word, ignoring the surrounding context.

As a coda, I must add that although Chapman et al. found that schizophrenics gave inappropriate strong associations, ironically, as I have shown elsewhere[4], samples of actual schizophrenic associational chaining often show highly unusual word associating, as in Brendan Maher's[5] example:

> To Wise and Company
> If you think that you are being wise to send me a bill for money I have already paid, I am in nowise going to do so unless I get the whys and wherefores from you to me. But where fours have been then fives will be and other numbers and calculations and accounts to your no-account no-bill noble nothing.

The associational chaining of *wise* with *whys* and *wherefores* with *where fours*, as well as *no bills* and *nobles* all seem highly unusual to me. In fact, I have never been able to elicit these pairs when giving word association tests.

Another pitfall for investigators who have not studied linguistics in any depth is to take the work of one scholar, latch on to one idea and then take that as the basis of their work. This is well exemplified in the works of Rodney Morice[6] and Philip Thomas.[7] Reading Chomsky's early works, both were impressed by Chomsky's emphasis on the fact that all human languages allow sentence embedding, Chomsky's term for subordinate clauses. Thus, first Morice and later Thomas presumed that sentence embedding was the heart of speech production. Being impressed by Chomsky's tree structure diagrams, Morice adopted them, thinking such a representation allowed him to count embedded sentences more scientifically, as in Figure 1.1. This figure shows that the subordinate clause 'who dated Tom' is derived, Chomsky's term, from an underlying sentence, 'the girl who dated Tom'.

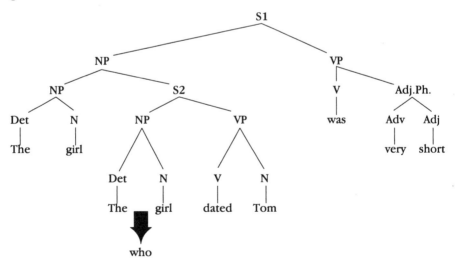

1. The girl was very short. The girl dated Tom.
                       ⇩ (Relative clause embedding)
1a. The girl who dated Tom was very short.

Figure 1.1: Tree structure diagram of an embedded sentence

Morice[8] went so far as to assume that 'One of the essential features of competent linguistic performance must be the production of sentences of appropriate syntactic complexity, complex enough to transmit relevant information ...' The problem here is that no metric of complexity has ever been devised as being necessary to encode any information. There is never just one way to express information of any sort. Very complex thoughts or complicated information can be expressed in a series of simple sentences which would show up as a series of simple, shallow Chomsky trees. Stylistically, this can be an exceedingly powerful mode of expression. In contrast, very mundane thoughts can be expressed in highly complex structures. This, in fact, defines the inflated speech of bureaucracy. Erroneous, even delusional thoughts may be expressed in complex sentences. Complexity of sentence structure is not isomorphic with complexity, truth, or even intelligence of thought. There is never just one way to express and develop any idea competently. Everything is paraphrasable, and every idea can be mapped upon variable syntactic structures for a variety of reasons.

For instance, one factor in whether or not to embed one sentence in another is to signal whether information being imparted is known to the hearer or not. For instance, consider van Dijk's[9] example:

1. Jack loves Mary. She's beautiful.
2. Jack loves Mary because she's beautiful.

In both of the above, the same information with the same degree of complexity is being imparted. In (1), the speaker is presupposing that the hearer did not know that Jack loved Mary. Therefore, this information is imparted in an independent sentence without subordinating the sentence giving the reason. On the other hand, (2) would be chosen if the hearer already knows that Jack loves Mary. Note that in (1), the hearer infers causation by the juxtaposition of the two propositions, whereas in (2) it is overtly stated. Each is equally complex, although (1) is labelled as two 'simple' sentences and (2) is labelled a 'complex' one. The so-called simple sentences in (1) are chosen if the speaker presumed that the hearer didn't know that Jack loves Mary, not because it represents simpler syntax. The so-called complex one is chosen because the speaker presumes the hearer does not know that Jack loves Mary. Complexity of thought and inferior linguistic competence do not necessarily have anything to do with the lack of sentence embedding in (1). Indeed, if the presuppositions that underly (2) are incorrect, and the hearer didn't know that Jack loved Mary, then the complex sentence is erroneous, so it is hardly an example of superior linguistic ability. Sometimes, as in this instance, purely semantic or informational requirements of the language determine whether or not embedding should take place.

Furthermore, even if it were true that schizophrenics did use less sentence embedding than non-schizophrenics in a given study, there may be extralinguistic factors for this. One is the matter of attentional deficit in schizophrenia. Because speech-disordered schizophrenics cannot subordinate their speech to a topic over as long a stretch as normal people can, they simply may not have the opportunity to embed sentences. That is, the schizophrenic is constantly veering to new topics, and introductory statements often do not contain much in the way of sentence embedding. That comes after, in the explanatory passages.

A prime rule of research is that all data must be accounted for. In language studies, since language itself comprises the data, all speech samples elicited in a study must be considered in any conclusions. Yet, Morice[10] says he parsed and drew his trees only on what he calls 'analysable sentences'. There is no mention of what made others unanalysable, why they couldn't be parsed at all, or why they couldn't be included in his analysis. However, it seems to me, their very unanalysability makes them important in any analysis and explanation of schizophrenic speech. Morice, after all, is trying to explain why this population speaks deviantly, so why throw out utterances which are so deviant that they don't fit on to a Chomsky tree? In sum, Morice 'proved' his point by disregarding any data that didn't fit his hypothesis. That isn't science. It's propaganda! Surprisingly, Philip Thomas[11] also advocates that one should simply ignore 'unanalysable' sentences. He explicitly says they should not be counted as part of the total. Yet their very occurrence, as well as their ratio to analysable sentences, is clearly important in discussing a population characterized by dysfluent speech. How can you characterize what dysfluencies are, much less understand their aetiology, if you throw out the very dysfluencies characteristic of the population? In any event, no scientist is given liberty to ignore data which do not happen to fit his or her theories. In research into language use, the language itself constitutes the data. Theories have to conform to data. Data can't be screwed into theories.

All this is not intended to suggest that linguists themselves always come up with the right theories or the right kinds of studies. As with other sciences, linguistics is littered with theories eventually found to be insufficient or just plain wrong. Corrections to theory are made by examining naturally produced or experimentally induced language and letting the data speak for themselves. Linguists, too, in the thick of their own conversations are usually as unconscious of what they're doing in encoding and decoding as is anyone else. However, when focusing on speech data, their special training in analysing language objectively allows them to bring to the fore and systematize the processes speakers and hearers undergo when producing speech, as well as to identify why certain forms are elicited and how they are perceived. This is not easy work. It often takes much difficult systematic analysis. Linguists have to record the speech they

are analysing so they can later pore over it and dissect it in order to find
relationships between what is said, the context of utterance, the nature of
deviation, if any, and the relationship between the way something is said
and what its meaning is. Sometimes linguists check hearers' or readers'
responses in order to discover how certain facets of language actually
work for speakers. Good linguistic analysis is never based upon the investigator's intuitions about how they think people will encode or decode a
stretch of language. Except for the chapter on schizophrenia, in this book
we shall be concerned with the structurally normal speech of clients and
what the clients inadvertently reveal about themselves by their use of
speech forms. The sources for judgments about such language use were
arrived at by careful analyses and dissecting of language elicited or
observed language samples.

Linguistic theories: new and old

Both pre-Chomskian structural linguistics and later transformational
theories presumed that syntax and semantics are separate fields of
language. However, more and more, linguists are finding the boundary
between them increasingly tenuous, showing that syntax cannot be
described without reference to semantics.[12] Chomskian Transformational-
Generative (hereafter, T-G) linguistics, and its descendants like 'The
Extended Standard Theory'[13] and 'Government-Binding' theories,[14] which
were certainly never the entire field of linguistics, have been perceived as
the cutting edge of the field by many, both in and outside of it. Some
linguists and non-linguists alike have been led to believe that linguistics is
an abstract description of language represented by arcane formulae and
diagrams.

T-G analyses were largely confined to a set of simplistic sentences like
'The farmer killed the duckling' or self-constructed sentences that virtually
nobody was likely to say, like 'He is the man to whom I wonder who knew
which book to give'.[15] Rather than listening to the speech around them
and trying to analyse what was going on in constructing it, many linguists
inspired by the Chomskian 'revolution' devoted themselves to discovering
what was and was not possible in grammars by constructing sets of
sentences from their own imaginations. They then 'determined' which
sentences were grammatical and which were not by their personal
intuitions. By looking at what was ungrammatical for them, they formu-
lated rules about what kinds of sentences human grammars could and
couldn't have, claiming this was how one could understand the human
mind. Most of these syntacticians based their conclusions not only on their
own made-up sentences, and their own intuitions, but on their own native
language, usually English. Early on, it became evident that the sentences
one linguist found acceptable another would find unacceptable, so
scholars were making pronouncements about what sentences 'in my

dialect' showed about the limits of human grammar. The absurdity of this still boggles my mind. How does one uncover the truth about the workings of an entire language on the basis of one's personal imagination in constructing sentences, especially when different people seem to have different ideas of what constitutes a grammatical sentence? How does one make judgments about the nature of the human mind and language if one considers only one of the thousands of languages spoken? And, of course, it is very easy to draw conclusions about language if one is willing to make up sentences which prove one's points, and not bother with those actually occurring sentences that do not.

To be fair, however, the transformationalists' practice of basing grammatical analyses on self-constructed sentences is part of their legacy from both nineteenth-century grammarians and some pre-Chomskian structuralist linguists.[16] Just as Chomsky at first wanted to describe a grammar used by an ideal speaker and listener, so did de Saussure and other early linguists think of actual speech as a falling away from some abstract ideal. De Saussure spoke of an abstract *langue* which was expressed often in debased form by *parole*. Chomsky used the terms *competence* vs. *performance* to indicate this difference between the ideal-ized entity and its realization in speech. However, language is something which is used, and used within contexts, and for various purposes. Far from being an abstract system that exists outside of speakers, a language, in my opinion, is the sum total of the grammars and lexicons that are in its speakers' minds. Speakers draw upon the system as they've learned it and, if need be, change it – because of the need either to express themselves or to present themselves as certain kinds of people. So long as they change it in a manner which other speakers can understand, so long as individual variation is small and confined to small parts of the overall system, then it will be perceived as being within normal limits. Another condition for normal language use is that it be subordinated to a topic that somehow fits the context of utterance. Verbal artists, of course, create their own topics and create deviations from usual usage in accordance with that topic. This ability of the individual to create new language forms is what makes language so flexible and why it changes so drastically over time.

Unfortunately, people do not speak individual sentences with no context, and they do form sentences to fit into discourses. Therefore, we can't explain language data on the basis of discrete sentences with no reference to context. Context itself is a broad concept, including the purpose of the discourse, and any other social factors that determine why a speaker would couch a certain idea one way and not another.

Linguists who rely on self-constructed sample sentences defend their practice on the grounds that the study of actual discourse is pragmatics, not linguistics. Fromkin,[17] for instance, derided my first analysis of schizo-phrenic speech. In that,[18] I claimed that schizophrenics broke linguistic rules on each level of language, giving samples of gibberish and word salads as well as disruptions in discourses. Fromkin retorted that the data I presented showed intact linguistic ability, although it showed that schizophrenics had problems with pragmatics. According to this view, then, linguistics and pragmatics, the way people actually use language, are separate scholarly disciplines, each with its own concerns and its own modes of analyses. In truth, there is no sharp dividing line between them. There is no linguistic element that is not used pragmatically and there are no pragmatic oral productions which are not composed of linguistic elements. For this reason, in this book, we analyse discourses except when discussing the use of culturally well-known proverbs in certain kinds of therapy. In that instance, we see that the cultural context of the proverb becomes a powerful backer of its meaning to clients trying to shake off culturally disapproved behaviours such as drug addiction.

There is another reason for rejecting the idea of a sentence-based grammar which purportedly generates only the sentences of a given language. This reason is purely historical. If a speaker used only those syntactic rules which generated sentences belonging to the language at any point in time, then the grammars of languages wouldn't ever change – but they do, and do drastically. Shakespeare's grammar is not our own, nor is Jane Austen's or even Sir Arthur Conan Doyle's. My students and I clearly differ on the acceptability and usage of certain syntactic usages. For instance, I would use a subjunctive after a verb like *recommend*, as in 'I recommend that he **get** here immediately.' Many of my students, who are a generation younger than I, would say 'I recommend that he **gets** here immediately', although those I taught 20 years ago used the subjunctive as I do. This example is historical. There are also regional and social dialectal variations within the same language! Clearly, syntax is not a fixed sentence-generating machine and it certainly is not a mathematical abstraction as Chomskian theorizing would have us believe. Indeed, an individual's syntax often offers potent insights into a patient's or client's world view. The only language I know of which seems to be a mere generation of utterances is in the disturbed narratives of some actively psychotic schizophrenics as shown in Chapter 5.

A simple instance of an abstract generative rule, is Chomsky's famous expression of the old grammatical idea that a sentence had a complete subject and a complete predicate by using the formula

S = NP + VP + (Adv) (meaning 'A sentence equals a noun phrase and a verb phrase')[19]

Fillmore,[20] however, early on noted that the idea 'subject of a sentence' is not just a syntactic relationship between a noun phrase and a verb phrase. It is also related to its verb by semantic relationships which are not overtly stated. In a ground-breaking essay, he showed that it isn't enough to speak of the subject of a sentence because each subject plays a certain role in conjunction to the verb. For instance, if someone says 'Max killed Oscar', then 'Max' takes on the meaning of [+agent]. He actively did the killing. If however, we say 'Oscar was killed', 'Oscar' is an object, but we don't know who or what killed Oscar, only that he was the recipient of some action or misfortune. If we say 'Oscar died', then Oscar is called a patient, one who underwent a process[21]and we are making no implications about who or what did him in. Perhaps he was 120 years old and his time had just come. The subject of *die* can never be an agent or a cause. It can only be a patient. The subject of *kill*, in contrast, is either an agent or cause, or, if the verb is in the passive (*was killed*), an object. Thus, verbs are marked, so to speak, by the roles[22] which their subjects may take.

An example of this is seen in the following anecdote. Billow et al.[23] recount a story about James Joyce and Dr Jung. Joyce was trying to refute Jung's diagnosis that Joyce's daughter was schizophrenic, saying 'She talks the way I write' to which Jung replied, 'But you dive, she falls.' Jung meant, of course, that Joyce controlled how he wrote, but his daughter had no control over her speech. That is why she was schizophrenic. Jung conveyed this meaning by his verb selection. *Dive*, by definition, has a feature of [+agent] on it. The one who dives, does it on purpose. *Fall* on the other hand is [−agent], meaning the one who falls usually does so by accident, not by his or her own agency.

There are other ways to encode sentences so as to avoid mention of agent or cause. In English we can use a 'dummy' subject like *it* or *there*, as in 'It's a bad day' or 'There was marijuana in my slippers'. In both of these sentences there is no mention of what or who is making the day bad or who put the marijuana in the slippers. Again, one who habitually uses such forms to the exclusion of using agents and causes is one who sees life as governed by capricious chance. Usually, such clients don't see their role in what happens to them. They don't see themselves or any of their actions as causes, so that their lives are just a bunch of incidents that happened to them. Later, when we meet Clive, we shall see such a patient.

Those who conceive of language as a system above and apart from usage, try to keep each level of language separate, thus imagining a pure level of phonology, another of syntax, and yet another of semantics. In actuality, as we shall see, it has become increasingly clear that there are fuzzy borders between categories, and that both syntax and semantics arise from the same underlying human situations and human perceptions. Scholars like Heine, Ruwet, and Langacker have produced an impressive body of work with data drawn from widely different languages.[24] As Langacker puts it 'It [cognitive grammar] contrasts with formalist approaches by viewing language as an integral facet of cognition (not as a separate "module" or "mental faculty").' He also points out that besides its semiological function of allowing thoughts to be symbolized by words, language has an interactive function, 'embracing communication, expressiveness, manipulation, and social communion'[25] and these are thoroughly intertwined when communicating.

These scholars, and others working in the functional/cognitive mode, show that both grammatical constructions and the way words are used are dependent upon the human experience of the world. To give a fairly trivial example, it is no accident that all languages seem to have grammaticized the idea of direct object, a noun that has something done to it. Humans regularly do things to other things. The construct of [verb + direct object] matches human activity. In like vein, humans extrapolate from their own bodies to inanimate objects, so that the word 'leg' in English and many other languages is used of furniture as well as one's own limb. All languages use analogous extensions in creating both syntactic systems and lexicons.

Langacker[26] shows how our experience of moving rapidly, running, gets encoded on to static situations in expressions like

> An ugly scar **runs** all the way from his knee to his ankle.
> The prices on this model run **from** about $18,000 all the way to $27,000...

In actuality the motion verb is used to describe static situations. Langacker says 'The sense of movement and directionality reflect the order in which a range of options ... are mentally accessed.' Note that each of these sentences has a parallel which shows a different scanning of the options:

> An ugly scar **runs** all the way from his ankle to his knee.
> The prices on this model **run** from about $27,000 down to $18,000.

It seems to me that we can use the verb 'run' in these situations because it evokes the usage of visually running our eyes over a scene. That is, we do with our eyes on a small scale what we do with our legs on a larger one, traversing a distance, and therein contains the similarity which allows us to use the same verb for both situations. Similarly, Langacker gives an example

> There's a cottage now and then through the valley.

He points out that 'A cottage is not the sort of thing that goes in and out of existence...Nor is anything described as moving, as suggested by the path phrase *through the valley*.' Technically, then, this should be nonsensical, but it is not. Rather, it evokes the way we see things as we are on a journey. Again, coherence is achieved and movement is given to a static situation by 'an active process of meaning construction'.[27] Again, it seems to me that such a process is possible because as the human moves through his or her environment, typically the view changes. We are very used to viewing from moving vehicles and also to viewing motion pictures, so we use those experiences in describing static situations that can't be taken in at one glance. That is, if there were but one cottage we wished to mention, we wouldn't do so using the imagery of a path or an adverbial phrase indicating things going in and out of view like 'every now and then', but we easily do so when describing more than one and their relationship to each other. A final example, one important to therapy, is that of verb tense. We naively believe that verb tense marks out time. It does, but it can also indicate point of view, as in

Ellen **was** writing furiously. **Tomorrow was** the deadline ...

Langacker says 'The incongruity of using *tomorrow* with a past tense verb signals ... Ellen's consciousness at the time of [her] writing.' In other words, we are made to feel as Ellen did as she was writing; we have moved into her mental space.[28]

Several researchers, like Chafe[29] and Miller[30] suggest that the phrase not the sentence, is the fundamental unit of grammar. I have long agreed, and, oddly enough, it was transformational grammars that convinced me. Working with sociolinguistics and discourse analysis, I noted early on that most interactions took place in phrases. For instance, if I enter the kitchen in the morning, my husband might just barely lift his eyes off the newspaper, but says to me 'All ready' and I know that the coffee is ready for me to pour and the toast is in the oven, done. In Chomskian terms, this would be taken as a sentence 'The coffee is all ready in the coffeemaker and the toast is done in the oven' with all the phrases that I can understand from the context having been deleted. That is, T-G syntax and its extended theories claim that the full sentence is first formed in the speaker's mind and then contextually obvious parts of the sentence are deleted.

The problem with such a view is that it overcomplexifies what has been said and understood. There is no reason for my husband first to create the entire sentence in his head and then delete the 'unnecessary' parts before uttering the phrase. In fact, one cannot even imagine language, which is unique to humans and exceedingly complex, to have evolved so that stand-alone phrases could be produced only by such acts of deletion from a deep structure sentence. It defies credulity. Grammarians convinced that the sentence is the basic unit of speech can save their theory only by positing such an unlikely psycholinguistic process as 'deletion' when faced with the phrases of ordinary conversation and even the fragments permissible in some kinds of writing.

What is more probable is that people form and utter only those phrases not recoverable from the context of utterance. Notice that phrases must be in proper grammatical form to be understood. Speakers don't usually say things like 'grammatical form to', or 'ran up the' or 'out of a' as informative chunks of language. Sentences are made up of phrases, and phrases can stand alone as basic meaning units. Phrases show specific structure like *the child I adopted, on the table, gone for the day, when Max comes*. And, as we shall see shortly, this phrasal construction is highly relevant to our memories and their activation. Certainly, phrases can be combined with other phrases to create sentences, but they can stand alone in the proper contexts. It's not for nothing that even Chomsky diagrammed his syntactic sentences as comprising phrase structures and that he defined *sentence* as being a 'noun phrase + verb phrase,' proceeding then to define how a noun phrase or a verb phrase is constructed.

This does not mean that sentences are not important units in grammar. Obviously, the very fact that phrases can be combined to form sentences show their importance. Halliday[31] shows how subjects and predicates can interact in a sentence to give meaning to the whole. He calls the subject the *theme*, the 'point of departure of the message' and the predicate is the *rheme*, what is said about the theme. However, as his own chapter on conversation shows, neither the subject nor the complete predicate need be stated overtly. Chafe[32] and Miller[33] both suggest that the sentence is more basic to written language than to spoken. That is not to say that spoken sentences aren't created orally. They are, but properly constructed phrases can also be used as complete units in speech, and often are.

Wallace Chafe[34] has done a good deal of work on how people recount events, showing that their phrasing matches the way their eye scans a scene. He has also correlated memories with phrasing. When he compared how people remembered a short movie six weeks after they first saw it, he found the 'content of intonation units [phrases] ... remaining virtually unchanged over a period of six weeks ... [but] organization of ... [phrases] ... into sentences shows little of the same stability'. That is, people remember phrases which encode what they saw, but not the actual sentences that those phrases were originally formed into. Apparently what gets remembered are the phrases, not the sentences. As a rule, people don't remember individual words out of phrases, either. This argues strongly for considering phrases as the basic units of both speech production and memory.

Chafe convincingly makes a case that, in speech as with vision, we are constrained in how much we can process at any one time. We move from one focal point to another, and this movement can be, and usually is, very rapid. In speech, the focal point is what he calls the **intonation unit**, which is a phrase. These are 'not produced in a continuous, uninterrupted flow but in spurts',[35] an observation Johnstone[36] agrees with and uses in her own analyses. These spurts are, as noted, phrases and are characterized by having one primary accent (or stress), but they may have secondary accents as well, as in (numbering Chafe's)

(1) a...And there were these twó wómen,
b...híking up ahéad of us[37]

(1)a and b comprise two intonation units, each with its own focal point. On grounds that would take us too far afield to discuss here, Chafe says that there is a 'one new idea constraint' which doesn't allow more than one new idea to be presented in an intonation unit. That is why the above was said as two separate units. In the above instance 'And there were these two women hiking up ahead of us', the phrases happen to comprise one sentence although sentencehood does not always follow by juxtaposed phrases. For example, consider

> Over the brídge
> Then on to ninéty-five

These were juxtaposed and were meant to be understood together as directions to get to the airport, but they certainly don't comprise a sentence. What does seem to happen always is that each phrase introduces no more than one unit of information, and combining phrases may or may not yield canonical sentences. When it does not, the phrases stand alone as independent structures of meaning. The written message, because it will be read in a variety of contexts, and is missing intonational cues, must include more structure; hence, in that medium the canonical sentence is preferred.

The intonation units, expressed in grammatically correct phrasal structures, represent the flow of information or thoughts as they come into consciousness. Then, if we wish, we can encode them into speech. We also decode others' speech by their intonation units. The units represent a chunking of information which allow us to understand as well as to present complex stories. We can keep in our consciousness only a very little information at one time, relative to the prodigious amount we have in our brains. As we speak, different information is activated and, Chafe claims, 'the number of different referents that can be active at the same time is very small, and ... any referent, unless it is refreshed, will quickly leave the active state'.[38] However, even if it isn't currently active, it still may be hovering nearby, which is why we can follow long discourses. Each piece of information we have is connected to many others which may be activated or semi-activated[39] as our focal points change, or as we notice items in the environment of speaking. If I understand Chafe correctly, then semi-active memories are those on 'standby' status and can easily be brought to the fore as our focal memories change.

Chafe also notes that information that is neither fully active nor demonstrably semi-active may still actually be stored at a shallower or deeper level. In other words, there are several states of activation and what transpires in an interaction will constantly change what is in which state. This theory accounts for the way an event in our visual purview, or a comment made by ourselves or another, makes us suddenly remember something. The constant flux in our focus also accounts for the annoying, but all too prevalent, forgetting of what we were just on the verge of saying. Another speaker mentions something else and our own activated memories become superseded by a newly activated one.

Two or more speakers in the same interaction may not have the same material brought to standby status, just below consciousness. Consider how often during a conversation, a participator suddenly says, 'Oh, that reminds me ...' Something just uttered or something in the environment has activated a memory. Then, further, what the person is reminded of may place that subject in the focal memory of the other interactor, and when this happens yet other memories are activated to some degree. What is important for therapy is that what the therapist says can guide the patient or client to bring uninstantiated material to focal or standby attention. It is this bringing up of certain matters to attention that causes repressed memories to surface.

Conversation and other speech become complicated also because we not only take account of the changing activation states of information in our own minds, but 'also attempt to appreciate parallel changes ... taking place in the minds of ... listeners'. Chafe states that

> Language is very much dependent on a speaker's beliefs about activation states in other minds. Such beliefs themselves constitute an important part of a speaker's ongoing, changing knowledge, and language is adjusted to accord with them.[40]

Our memories are encoded in language, for the most part, and are brought to the surface, that is, instantiated, by verbal interactions. Since the meanings of words include the emotions an individual associates with them, the emotions themselves, even if long buried, are instantiated along with the phrase or word. That's why therapists have to keep tissues handy for their clients. The routines and motor experiences that have become attached to certain words are also part of their meaning. Part of the meaning of *chair* is the position we assume when on it.

Chafe's theory, one which agrees with other researchers on activation of memory by scholars like Baars,[41] and Reason,[42] also explains the phenomenon of buried memories which become recalled in psychotherapy. Despite the attacks on buried memories in recent years, at least in the United States court systems, it seems possible, even certain, that some memories remain inactive for years, if a certain topic is not discussed or otherwise refreshed, until questions or topics brought up in conversation allow them to be activated. Since emotion is associated with events in memory, memories may be buried so as to avoid the pain that is relived on activation. Given the nature of therapy and its emphasis on questioning and recall, buried memories can be expected to surface. The theory of memory activation makes as much sense in explaining painful buried memories as does a theory which claims that therapists have 'planted' memories in patients' minds.

Chafe's discoveries about the activation states is also highly pertinent to understanding the chaining quality of some psychotic speech. Consider the following schizophrenic response to the question of what colour a certain chip was:

1. Looks like clay, sounds like gray, take you for a roll in the hay, hay day, May Day, help. I need help

The first phrase was on target. The chip was clay-coloured, but the rest were activated phrases associated by connections both with the syntactic form used and the phonological shape of the words. Finally, the semantic features of one word in the inappropriately evoked rhyming sequence, *hay day, Mayday*, evoked the plea for help. The very fact that the elicited rhymes were put into phrases fortifies Chafe's theory, and his theory explains why such chains occur.

In non-psychotic people, what gets activated in memory depends on the topic of the utterance. In speech-disordered schizophrenics activation can occur with words related by sound or by meaning alone, ungoverned by any relationship to a topic. Interestingly, the first part of such speech disorder typically does fit the context. It is as the patient continues to talk that he or she activates inappropriate phrases. Many scholars[43] now concur that there is an **executive function** in the brain which helps select words and phrases appropriate to the topic at hand, but that this executive fails in schizophrenia, accounting for activations of phrases that aren't subordinated to the topic. It may well be, however, that the very instantiating of memories not specific to the task at hand may still yield important clues to traumatic events in a schizophrenic's life, although at others times, they may just be intrusive. For instance, the following two narratives were elicited from schizophrenics who were asked to describe a short video-story they had just seen. The first shows intrusions from the speaker's desire to see her brother, but the second one hints strongly at the patient's memories of being abused at the hands of men as well as to a remembered failure of a brother in discharging his task of watching over a girl. Since there was neither a brother or even a male playmate shown in the video, nor was there anything about anyone who was supposed to be watching over the little girl, we can suppose that these are memories accessed by certain situations in the video. Buying ice cream is equated with buying a candy bar; the scenes with the mother and father recall an event concerning a brother; the father (who actually gives the child money for ice cream in the video) reminds the patient of men who use women. It must be stressed that there was no abuse of any sort shown in the video-story, which was a charming vignette of an obviously loved child who wanted an ice cream cone.[44]

1. What do you want me to say? I saw my brother Gene. He says he said I buy the things that I wanted. I saw a little girl who wanted ice cream. Today you have to

pay for it but today she paid for it. I want Gene to come visit me soon at 1:30 and I saw a little girl with the baby and her father's gonna be home an and oh yeah an [hehe] my mother loves me [aw hehe]. I don't know what I want to say. Can I stop now?[45]

2. Okay. I was watchin' a film of a little girl and um s bring back memories of things that happened to uh people around me that affected me durin' the time when I was livin' in that area and uh she jus' went to the store for candy bar and by the time ooh of course her brother who was supposed to be watchin' wasn't payin' much attention he was blamed for and I didn't think that was fair the way the way they did that either so that's why I'm kinds like askin' yah could we just get together for one big party or something ezz it hey if it we'd all in which is in not they've been here so why you jis now discoverin' it. You know they've been men will try to use you every time for everything he wants so ain't no need and you tryin' to get upset for't that's all that's all.[46]

Notice that in both of the above discourses, there is no orderly presentation of phrases that would correspond to an orderly scanning of the scenes in memory. This is typical of schizophrenic narration and fits well into other language symptoms, such as gibberish and word salads which show linguistic elements not ordered correctly into larger units.[47] However, the memories triggered by events, although not as 'orderly' as in normal people, still show the same process of being reminded by what is said or seen, of older memories or newer ones, being brought to the fore. Of course, videotapes are not necessary to access memories. A therapist's questions will do. What these findings mean to therapists is that they must listen carefully to the patient's or client's speech and note statements that can be questioned and that may lead to deeper discussion.

Such examples show how lexical and grammatical choices mirror our experiences. Current linguistics unabashedly views language as a mirror to thought and physical processes, such as scanning a scene. Where once I insisted[48] upon keeping language and thought separate in analyses, I now see that newer understandings of the cognitive underpinnings of language[49] promise insights into the nature of thought disorder, for instance, in schizophrenia. They also promise insights into understanding the narratives told by clients who are not psychotic.

This does not mean that language and thought are one and the same, however. For one thing, the same thought may be expressed in hundreds of different languages, so it can't be directly equated with any particular language form. For another, one has to have a certain thought before deciding what words and phrasing one is going to use in expressing it. That is, the thought is parent to the speech. Moreover, even within a language, the same thought may be expressed in alternative ways. Sometimes the very alternative the speaker has chosen in which to express a given idea yields clues to his or her underlying thoughts. We shall see this clearly in Chapter 6, 'Telling a life'.

Using language

Language is not simply a system of communication. It is used for sundry purposes and palpable effects. There is no aspect of human endeavour which is untouched by language.[50] Every test we take, every bit of knowledge we garner, the ways we relate to others, the recipes we decide to try out, the sports we play, our humiliations and our feelings of pride, the people who are kept 'in their place', and the ones who are privileged, all are mediated through language. Our societies run on language. We bond with others through language, or we feel separated from others through language. To be human is to be a language user. There is no way to consider any human institution or interaction without considering also the language that was or was not used in creating it.

We show our personal identities by the choices we make in speaking: the pronunciations we adopt, the forms of sentences, the selection of words, and even our voice quality itself, whether it is gentle or strident, hesitant or assured.[51] We stock our prodigious memories in language and we retrieve them by someone else's – or our own – words.[52] We even create our own selves and protect our own egos through the way we narrate our own lives to ourselves and to others.[53] Most important for us, here, is that all mental health therapy is done through language: the topics that get raised, the questions answered, the memories instantiated through talk, and the underlying motives and meanings of a client's tales. Because speech is so ubiquitous, and because people usually employ it with so little conscious preparation, they are not aware of the truly awesome complexities of how even ordinary speech is produced and understood. Chafe[54] describes the subconsciousness of linguistic processing as

> linguistic form ... located in a pane of glass through which ideas are transmitted from speaker to listener. Under ordinary circumstances language users are not conscious of the glass itself, but only of the ideas that pass through it. The form of language is transparent, and it takes a special act of will to focus on the glass and not the ideas. Linguists undergo a training that teaches them how to focus on the glass, but fluent users of a language focus their consciousness only on what they are saying.

And, we might add, what they are understanding. We think of understanding as a passive and automatic process although, as we have just seen in Langacker's examples, it often involves our imagining ourselves to be in certain situations, such as travelling along a path or making a parallel between an activity like running and scanning a static situation. It may also involve our putting ourselves in someone else's mind, as in Ellen's writing because 'Tomorrow **was** the deadline.' In actuality, understanding is even more of a highly mentally active process. First we must chunk the stream of sound into separate words, then chunk the words into phrases. Next, we must figure out the relation of the phrases to each other, and match the whole to the context. To make it even more complex, context includes the immediate linguistic context as well as the general cultural context, the relative social statuses between conversationalists or, if written language is the object, the genre of the writing, the authority or lack thereof of the author, and so on. In other words, we don't passively understand. We actively construe. We get glimpses into the process only when we fail to understand and then become aware of our struggle to do so.

When language is not understandable, we blame the locus of our misunderstanding on the speaker's failure. How we view that failure will determine how we treat the speaker. If we view it as an unintentional slip, we politely try to repair, saying, 'Oh, do you mean X?' or the like. If we view it as a refusal to co-operate in treatment, we may decide to punish the patient in some way. If we view it as a client's trying to give voice to unacceptable ideas, we see our task as trying to evoke those ideas from the client's subconscious. If we see it as uninterpretable gibberish from a drug-induced state or a dementia, we don't try to interpret it at all. Language is so bound up with the way we behave towards each other that our interpretations of others' speech often has important and even severe consequences.

The key word here is *interpretation*. At no point is language necessarily isomorphic with meaning. That is, there is no necessary one-to-one correspondence between message and meaning. How an utterance is constructed and what it actually means are never necessarily identical. Messages may mean more, less, or something different from the sum of their parts: 'a Venetian blind' and 'a blind Venetian' refer to wholly different entities, as do 'the savings count' and 'count the savings.' 'It's hot here' can mean 'Please turn on the air conditioner' or 'Open a window, for God's sake' or 'I'm going to the beach.' 'Yeah, great' as a response if said with the tone that embodies sarcasm means 'that's not great' and, at the same time, expresses scorn for the first speaker or the speaker's expressed view. If said enthusiastically, it means 'that *really* is great' and expresses admiration for the first speaker.

Messages may mean nothing beyond the fact that a message is required in certain social situations. Politeness routines like 'Hello there' are essentially so devoid of meaning that, in passing, one so greeted might just respond with 'Fine, and you?' which relates to the original statement only that it is a recognized response for a greeting. Similarly, as a greeting in passing 'How are you?' is not a real request for information, although, in the therapeutic situation, it may well be the opener for the session. That is, in one context, a phrase has no real meaning beyond pure social recognition, but in another, the same phrase is both an invitation and a springboard to hearing about the client's problems.

Bureaucratic language is notorious for the emptiness of its phrasing, as is much scholarly writing which, when distilled, means far less than its pomposity would lead one to believe. For instance

It seems the simplest way to show the generality of the categorization problem is by showing that no uncategorized population may be specified such that only one categorization device is available for categorizing the population's personnel.[55]

Apparently, what this means is that every group can be categorized in more than one way. By phrasing in such a loquacious manner, however, the speaker is also cueing the reader that this is a scholarly statement, a product of wide observation and deep thought and not just an ordinary observation. It is a way of claiming special intelligence and superiority. So, the passage means both that every group can be categorized in more than one way and that the speaker has an extraordinary intellect. It's easy to make fun of such passages, but most scholars resort at least occasionally to verbal pyrotechnics to prove their intellectual acuity. Indeed, editors and other scholars often demand such language as proof that the writer or speaker is not merely stating known mundane facts. The novelty of the expression itself hides the readily available truism of the observation.

The fact that language is not isomorphic between message and meaning also means that it is potentially highly ambiguous. Context is essential for disambiguation, so all language is context-bound. This, of course, creates problems for the therapist, who must concentrate not only on the therapeutic context, but must often recreate the client's mental context. Chomsky's desire to create a context-free grammar which would generate all the sentences of a language was doomed to failure because, excepting examples in scholarly tomes, all language is produced in a context and is interpretable within that context. Moreover, context itself is not simply the circumstance or place of utterance, but includes what the interactants presume each other knows because of previous interactions and the sharing of a common culture. It also includes recognition of the social status and professional standing of each interactant. All these factors have bearing on both what is said and how it is to be interpreted. The latter also depends upon the interpreter's beliefs about why the other has said what he or she has said. Later, in our discussion of a client, Helena, we shall see that a statement that she made in order to show how she was mistreated was apparently misconstrued by her psychiatrist as a form of bragging. The results were disastrous for the client and, insofar as losing a paying client inconveniences a psychiatrist, didn't lead to a happy outcome for him either. Because the same forms take on different meanings in different social and linguistic contexts, language is infinitely flexible and able to yield new meanings, but it also takes thoughtful inter-pretation.

It is interesting that Noam Chomsky tried to create a context-free grammar when grammar itself out of context is ambiguous. Every syntactic construction may be used for several functions. Chomsky himself did note the ambiguity of sentences like 'Max decided on the boat', which can mean 'Max decided something while he was on the boat' or 'Max decided to buy a particular boat.' *On the boat* can either be a prepositional phrase indicating location, or the *on* may be part of the two-part verb *decide on*.[56]

Mutual understanding, then, is not an automatic matching process. Rather, speakers have to compare all the words and the syntax they use with the context. Part of the process includes what they think is in the minds of their co-speakers. Typically, a speaker thinks co-speakers put the same value on each word that the speaker does. Speakers assume that the co-speaker can fill in what wasn't overtly said because of the assumption that all are sharing the same context. If a speaker doesn't assume that another shares the same context, then the speaker fills in that information, or runs the risk of being misunderstood. Of course, if the speaker persists in retelling what the hearer already knows, then the speaker is a bore with all the social consequences attendant upon that label. Speaking skilfully entails constant judgments about the context. As indicated above, context includes everything from the relative social statuses of the speakers, to the perceived intention of what has been said, to how intimate the speakers are, to the environment and locale of speaking. Hanks[57] puts it well: language is saturated with context.

Normally, this actually creates an advantage because it means that anyone can take a word already in the language, or a phrase or a sentence, and by putting it in a new context, a hearer or reader will be able to construe a new meaning. Thus, a speaker may use his or her old language to say new things. New words can even be constructed by speakers and, if sufficient context is given, the hearer can assume what they mean. Comprehension is a matter of joint production between speaker and hearer, and, as we shall see in Chapter 3, between therapist and client.[58]

Linguists have long recognized that each speaker has an idiolect,[59] his or her own set of language rules and vocabulary meanings. Johnstone[60] emphasizes the individuality of speech usage as did Quirk and Svartvik,[61] discussed below. Indeed, tacitly, at least, linguists have long noted the individual variation in using language, referring to our **idiolects**[62] **as well as dialects** in our language.

Hanks,[63] among others who study actual interactions, emphasizes that although there is a large common code, the same language differs in many respects from person to person.[64] What a word or phrase means is highly variable according to the experiences of the person using it.[65] The routines[66] associated with a word can also become part of its meanings, so that part of the meaning of ice-skate for a New Englander like me is the gliding in the cold brightness of the frozen starlight at night. Beck[67] points out that the motor habits associated with a word are also part of its definition. The way we seat ourselves and then sit on a chair helps to define its concept and 'help to subtly distinguish chairs from other objects that can be sat on.' It has occurred to me that the philosophical conundrum presented to me in my first college philosophy class, 'What constitutes the chairness of a chair' is solvable by recognition that our bodily motion and subsequent position helps define what *chair* is.

Johnstone[68] stresses that, although speakers of a language share much language, each still uses some parts of it idiosyncratically. Even when people share the same word stocks, what the individual items mean may be affectively different from one speaker to the next. If I say 'She is a strong, intelligent woman who knows how to get ahead,' I am admiring her strength and perseverance, but if a person doesn't share my view of female power, the same utterance might mean she is a harridan or a shrew. The belief systems of speakers determine the full affective and emotional meanings they derive from the same words. This can become very important in therapeutic situations. What does the client mean by his or her word or phrase choice? It may be quite different from what another client means or from what the therapist presumes. Joint defining of key words is often very much in order and may be an important part of therapy, especially when we consider, as we did when discussing Chafe's work, how memories are instantiated by words.

Linguistic acceptability

It has already been emphasized that all linguistic forms are polysemous. That is, everything can mean many things. Context, be it physical, social, cultural, historical, or the result of personal experience, is the ultimate determiner of meaning. Hanks[69] makes the point that *literal meaning is the product of context* [italics mine]. Speakers, because of distraction or pathology, may make errors. A normal error typically involves a word or structure close to the mark and is recoverable by matching it to the context. A normal slip might involve substituting one word in a set for another, such as saying 'today' instead of 'tomorrow'. Or, it might involve a transposition of two sounds, so that 'prune the roses' turns into 'rune the proses'. Also, when confronted with their error, normal people recognize it, but psychotics often show no awareness even when you point it out to them. These remarks should not be taken to mean that all psychotics produce deviant speech. They do not, but when they do, the error is usually definably different from normal error.[70]

Researchers or therapists working with psychotic populations, expecting speech deviations, may interpret normal error or idiolectal variation in word meaning as being schizophrenic. The same phenomenon will be interpreted quite differently according to our judgments about the speaker. For instance, conversants may think that non-prestige speakers are speaking in a fragmented, disjointed style, while perceiving prestige speakers as uttering full sentences, when, in reality, both groups speak in phrases. How you interpret someone's speech and how you evaluate it cause you to get quite different meanings from the same phenomena. Docherty et al.,[71] for instance, in trying to refine diagnoses between schizophrenia and mania by using language criteria, mistakenly took several sentences with no errors or normal dysfluencies, and termed them deviant and as 'communication failures'. However, the statements they present are completely comprehensible. For instance, they give as a sign of pathology:

1. I'm hoping they don't get caught up in some of the ills of our life, of our society.
2. It seems so, you know, this, that, or the other.
3. Those people don't belong on the earth. God will get them.
4. I used to sit in the café, have something to eat and just **glare** out in the night.

Their objection to (1) is that 'ills of our life, of our society' is a vague reference. Surely, it is a trite one, but hardly pathological. Utterance (2) is actually a creative way of indicating that something is wishy-washy. I may not like the semantic import of (3), but it is expressed in normal language. Docherty et al. single out the word *glare* as being deviant in (4), but there is nothing pathological or even wrong about it. *The Random Dictionary* (2nd edn) gives as one of the meanings of *glare*: 'a fiercely or angrily piercing stare'. Unless Docherty et al. had information to the contrary, then (4) is a perfectly ordinary usage when describing one's anger.

Recognizing variability within individual language stocks, grammarians like Quirk and Svartvik,[72] before deciding whether or not a structure was acceptable (normal) for other speakers, devised what they called 'acceptability tests' to discover whether or not different speakers found certain constructions acceptable in the sense of 'belonging to the English language'. In these tests, they were not testing for English grammatical forms which are socially disvalued but are clearly part of English, like 'I ain't got none'. Rather, they used sentences which they knew to have variable forms like 'He isn't but he claims so.' Some British native speakers found this perfectly acceptable, but others had to change it to 'He isn't but he claims to be.' Notice these are not idiolectal differences, but differences that occur over a large set of speakers. Similarly, whereas some felt no violation of syntax with 'The old man found his son a wife', others did, preferring instead 'The old man found a wife for his son.'

Such minor differences between speakers do not hinder communication, and often aren't even noticed in the thick of conversation, but they do show individual variation in syntactic rules. Also, the variations in each instance are not wholly different from each other and the differences centre on synonymous phrases. *So* is a pro-word often used to indicate 'go back to the last verb phrase and fill it in here mentally' and *to be* is used the same way. For instance, I can say 'He is very poor and *so* is Jack.' The *so* means 'is very poor'. I can also say, 'He is very poor, and Jack claims *to be*.' The *to be* also means 'is very poor.' *So* and *to be* are both used for the same function, so it is not surprising that different speakers habitually use *so* where others use *to be*.

The variation between 'The old man found his son a wife' vs. 'The old man found a wife for his son' matches the normal variation in indirect objects as in 'The old man poured his son some tea' vs. 'The old man poured a cup of tea for his son.' The indirect object construction itself involves only a few verbs and different dialects or groups of speakers allow it in some instances where others wouldn't. For instance, I often ask 'Reach *me* a glass, please' whereas I am continually surprised to discover that most of my students over the years only allow 'Reach a glass *for me*, please.' Apparently my usage is idiolectal, but it does clearly mean 'get a glass for me', even to those who would never say it the way I do. They understand it with no trouble. Idiolectally or dialectally different speakers allow certain forms to be included in the set of verbs which can take indirect objects. There is a small difference among speakers, however, as to which verbs can or can't. This kind of variability is normal in language and is a product of the fact that we all have to learn our language for ourselves. Individual variation typically can be explained by other, related forms in the language. There are enough similarities so we can see how these came to be differentiated between different groups of speakers.

Pathological error is far wider of the mark than normal errors, and also than normal idiolectal or dialectal variation is. Consider

> 2. After John Black has recovered in neutral form of life, the honest bring back to life doctor's agents must take John Black through making up design meaning straight neutral underworld shadow tunnel.[73]

Although this is clearly deviant and incomprehensible as well, it does show some normal structure. It opens with a recognizable introductory adverbial clause *After John Black has recovered in neutral form of life*. The subject, ... *doctor's agent* comes before the main verb *must take* and its object *John Black* is in the correct position. The verb forms are both correct in their use of auxiliaries and endings: *has recovered* and *must take*. There is a recognizable prepositional phrase *through ... tunnel*. The problem is that no structural markers tell us how to interpret such chains as *making up design meaning straight underworld shadow* and the words themselves can't be construed together on the basis of any of their semantic features. The patient seems to be trying to talk about recovering from an illness (his own?) and after this recovery the doctors will make him go through a tunnel. Perhaps *a neutral form of life* is life after mental illness. Given the insufficiency of syntactic markers, and the difficulty in interpreting the words strung together, all this is pure conjecture on my part. Like the associative chaining seen in (2) above, we see lexical items put together that don't seem to be obeying a topic.

Schizophrenics often produce deviant syntax, much of it like aphasic speech or even massive amounts of slips of the tongue,[74] but there is one deviation that I have seen only in schizophrenics, and that is leaving out the object of a verb without any prior context showing what its object is, as in 'Do you have?' 'I have.' Both of these were uttered by a speech disordered schizophrenic, one whose speech was so disorganized that she produced long chains of gibberish. There was no prior noun that could have been understood as the object of *have*, so this was deviant, not a product of ellipsis.

The seriousness of this can be seen if we consider the special relationship between verbs and their objects. The [verb + object] relationship is very strong, stronger than the link between subject and verb. Just think of how many idioms are in the form of [verb + object] *pull X's leg, sell X down the river, bought the farm, kicked the bucket, take a leak.* To my knowledge there isn't one idiom in the form of [subject + verb] if the verb requires an object. Also, we have pro-words that substitute for [verb + object], like *so did* and *do, too*, as in

Mary ate pork chops and so *did* Jack.
Mary loves ice cream sodas and *so do* I.

The *so did* means 'ate pork chops' and the *so do* means 'loves ice cream sodas'. There is no pro-word that stands for the subject and verb as a unit.

Schizophrenics may also sever the strong relationship with *the* and a noun. *The* is a noun determiner. That is, it must be completed by a noun, as in '**the** grape ice **cream**' A schizophrenic, recounting a narrative to me, for instance, said 'I gave him *the* and carried it home.' *The* marks the beginning of a noun phrase, and *have* used as a full verb marks the beginning of a [verb + noun phrase]. In other words, schizophrenic speech can become so disintegrated that it actually violates the structure of the phrase, which, we have already seen, is the basic unit of production and of meaning.

Syntax and point of view

We have seen that language resides in the minds of individual speakers and is intimately bound up with cognition and experiences. Enough is shared so that speakers of the same language can understand each other, but there are also individual differences. What interests us here is the way individual speakers draw upon the resources of the language in accordance with the way they perceive the world or the way they want the world to perceive them. It is also interesting to look at how people show their individual points of view, their emotional involvement, by their choice of language forms. We have also seen that the subject of a sentence may carry meanings like 'agent', 'cause', 'instrument' or 'patient'.

Our interest in the relationships such as that between a subject and its verb is how people use them. Usually one has a choice when encoding an event. One can choose verbs with agents or verbs with patients. For instance, in encoding a narrative or simply conversing, some people frequently use verbs with agents or causes as their subjects. Their sentences take the form of 'I did this' and 'I did that', thus taking responsibility for what has happened, or at least showing an awareness of cause and effect in a usually orderly world. Others, however, avoid agents as much as is linguistically possible, saying 'This occurred,' or 'That occurred' or 'This happened to me', 'That happened to me.' Notice that the person who says 'That happened *to me*' is also expressing that he or she is a victim. Such speakers may also choose the passive verb form over the active one in order to avoid mentioning agents or causes, as in 'He was harmed' rather than 'I harmed him'. In sum, they choose verbs that don't allow agents as subjects or they use a syntactic structure that allows the agent not to be expressed.

A psychologist colleague of mine asked, 'So I notice that a patient doesn't use agents. What do I do?' I myself am not a therapist, so I don't feel qualified to do more than point out the problem, but, if we think of therapy partly as learning to use language differently, orally and in our thoughts, then why not act like a teacher? Ask 'Who did that?' 'Where did that marijuana come from? Who put it there?' 'How did that happen?' 'Who made it happen?' 'What was used so that happened?' and the like.

In other words, as much as possible make the client or patient re-encode using agents and causes. This should help accustom them to thinking in terms of agents, causes and instruments as bringing certain things to pass. Hanks[75] claims that 'If a feature of context ... is encoded, then speakers using the language are **habituated** to take notice of the corresponding aspect of context.' If agency and cause become habitual, then a client becomes more attuned to seeing their own contribution to situations.

Adverbials are also strong encoders of points of view. If a client ties together events with phrases starting with *consequently, therefore, because, that led to ..., on account of* .... and the like, then they are showing that they understand the reasons behind events, or that there are reasons behind events. This action produces that result. They may be ascribing cause and event erroneously. For instance, if someone says, 'I lost my job because I was always late to work', he or she has a good grip on cause and effect. If, however, they say 'I lost my job because aliens took over my boss's brain' they are probably ascribing cause erroneously. In other words, just because someone does utilize adverbials and similar phrases that show causation, that doesn't mean necessarily that he or she has seen the event properly. If the client is lucid enough and the therapist feels that the ascribed causation is probably not valid, he or she could try to elicit other probable causes from the client. That is, a discussion of alternative causes can be initiated. Again this habituates a client to think of likely causes.

Some clients, often the same ones who don't use agents or causes, rarely use words that indicate that one event is caused by another. Instead, they rely on adverbials like *all of a sudden, out of the blue, with no warning, can you believe it,* or *you'll never believe it but . . .* For such clients, like ones who don't choose to name agents or causes, things just happen to them. The clients don't cause them to happen, and neither does anything else. The world is simply a fickle place. We shall see this with Meg and Esther in Chapter 6. If at all possible, such clients have to be gently pushed towards seeing cause and effect, towards using words like *because* and *consequently.* The therapist can ask questions like, 'What were you doing when that happened?' 'What was going on when that happened?' Or, 'What was going on just before that happened?' 'Why were you doing it?' 'Do you like doing that?' 'Don't you resent having to do that?' or whatever questions seem appropriate. The attempt here is to get the client or patient to see that events are connected. Sometimes things do happen out of the blue, but sometimes they do not. Kuno[76] develops the interesting proposition that the syntax chosen for a given sentence corresponds to the perspective of the speaker. Kuno[77] explains that

> speakers unconsciously make the same kind of decisions that film directors make about where to place themselves with respect to the events and states that their sentences are intended to describe ...

He describes such decisions as being describable in terms of empathy. Kuno shows, for instance, that

John hit Bill

is an unmarked empathy condition. It projects an objective view. In this encoding no particular empathy is being shown either to John or to Bill. It merely states that John, the agent, initiated the hitting and that Bill has received it. However, if a speaker refers to John as Bill's brother, then

Bill's brother hit him (*him = Bill*)

shows more empathy with Bill than with his brother. Kuno observes that it 'seems commonsensical' that the possessive chosen, here *Bill's brother*, would be used to refer to John only 'when the speaker has placed himself closer to Bill than his brother'. This is because the brother is seen in this construction only through his relationship with Bill, not as an independent person. In other words, Bill's relationship is more important than the independent characterization of calling John by name. I think here, too, by emphasizing the sibling relationship, one is emphasizing that it is not a good thing when one's brother hits one, and that affects the empathy felt towards Bill. If the speaker says

Bill was hit by John

he or she has identified with the subject of the passive verb, in this instance, Bill. The passive form signalled by *was hit* and encoding the agent with *by John* is a transformation from the more usual active: John hit Bill. Kuno[78] observes that the passive in general makes us feel more empathy towards the new subject, here, Bill. Why go to the trouble of creating a passive, making the object the new subject, unless one wishes to draw attention to him? To Kuno, that attention is empathy. Svartvik[79] claims that is actually quite rare to have passives with one word agents thrown to the end of the sentence as it is here with *by John*. More typically, the *by John* would be left out. Since it hasn't been, leaving it in emphasizes the agent, John, and since hitting is pejorative when it has both a human subject and object, then one is emphasizing blame on John and, with that, empathy for Bill. Another empathy condition occurs in

Bill was hit by his brother

This is also a passive which shows empathy for Bill, but this seems to relate to an overriding empathy condition: that if you do not directly name someone whose name is presumably likely to be known to you, then you are showing empathy for the one whose name you did use.

Chimombo and Roseberry[80] show that one can use *this* or *that* to show emotional closeness or distance. They give as an example 'This was a very naughty thing to do' when telling a story to a child. It seems to me also that *that* refers to a less immediate circumstance, e.g. 'That bothers me' as opposed to 'This bothers me.' *That* may not be in view and the event is over, whereas *this* indicates the here and now. If one is holding an article of clothing, one might say 'I love this blouse' but if another has it on, then one says 'I love that blouse.' Given the distancing function of *that*, one can note in a therapeutic setting when the speaker uses *this* or *that* to indicate emotional closeness or distance, or to indicate how vivid something still is in the speaker's mind.

Haiman[81] carries such analyses, those by Kuno and by Chimombo and Roseberry, even further. His work on both sarcasm and politeness have led him to show how language may be alienated from the emotions that produced it. He avers that

> Speakers using language in general are *eo ipso* alienated from the emotions they describe. Once they control them sufficiently to use language, they are not merely expressing them but also describing them; no longer merely, or even primarily, participants, they have become observers and exorcists of their emotional turmoil.

Throughout his book, Haiman[82] also shows that many languages, English included, have grammaticalized forms which show self-alienation. The reflexive used in sentences like

The judge removed *himself* from the case
Pull *yourself* together
I don't know how they live with *themselves*[83]

indicates a divided self, as if one is two people and one can observe and control the other. We see this also in expressions like 'Don't pat yourself on the back.' What is interesting is that older English did not have a reflexive of this kind and many languages extant do not. Haiman sees this as self-alienation, a particularly modern condition.

In sum

This chapter has taken us on a difficult ride through the thickets of linguistic theory. It showed the special role of the linguist in evaluating and understanding all situations dependent upon language. It espouses the view that language is not some abstraction apart from general human cognition. The basic unit of spoken language is the phrase, not the sentence, and the way people join together phrases reflects the way they are scanning what they're talking about. Language resides in the minds of all its speakers, but the way that speakers utilize language forms varies in accordance with the way they view the world or a particular segment of it. People can avoid responsibility, for instance, by habitually phrasing sentences by not using agents as subjects. People also reflect their empathies by their choice of linguistic forms. This chapter has also shown that both understanding language and producing it are active processes. Subsequent chapters will show how the ideas presented here can be turned into practice for the therapist.

Notes

1. Capps L, Ochs E (1995) Constructing Panic: The Discourse of Agoraphobia. Cambridge, Mass.: Harvard University Press, 66–7.
2. Chaika E (1974) A linguist looks at 'schizophrenic' language. Brain and Language 1: 257–76.
3. Chapman L, Chapman J, Daut R (1976) Schizophrenic inability to disattend from strong aspects of meaning. Journal of Abnormal Psychology 85: 35–40.
4. Chaika E (1990) Understanding Psychotic Speech: Beyond Freud and Chomsky. Springfield, Illinois: Charles C Thomas, 32.
5. Maher B (1972) The language of schizophrenia: a review and an interpretation. British Journal of Psychiatry 120: 4–17.
6. Morice RD, Ingram JC (1982) Language analysis in schizophrenia: diagnostic implications. Australian and New Zealand Journal of Psychiatry 16: 11–21.
7. Thomas P (1994) A Manual for the Brief Syntactic Analysis, mimeo; Thomas P, Leudar I (1995) Syntactic processing and communication

disorder in first-onset schizophrenia. In Sims A (ed) Speech and Language Disorders in Psychiatry. London: Gaskell, 96–112.

8. Morice R (1995) Language impairments and executive dysfunction in schizophrenia. In Sims A (ed) Speech and Language Disorders in Psychiatry. London: Gaskell, 61.

9. van Dijk T (1988) News as Discourse. Hillsdale, NJ: Lawrence Erlbaum, 60.

10. Morice R (1995) Language impairments and executive dysfunction in schizophrenia. In Sims A (ed) Speech and Language Disorders in Psychiatry. London: Gaskell, 58.

11. Thomas P (1994) A Manual for the Brief Syntactic Analysis 5, 28.

12. Heine B, Claudi U, Hünnemeyer F (1991) Grammaticalization: A Conceptual Framework. Chicago: University of Chicago Press; Heine B (1997) Cognitive Foundations of Grammar. New York: Oxford University Press; Duffley PJ (1992) The English Infinitive. English Language Series. New York: Longmans; Levin B (1993) English Verb Classes and Alternations. Chicago: University of Chicago Press; Chafe W (1968) Idiomaticity as an anomaly in the Chomskyan paradigm. Foundations of Language 4: 109–27; McCawley J (1968) Lexical insertion in a transformational grammar without deep structure. Papers from the Fourth Regional Meeting of the Chicago Linguistic Society: 71–80.

13. Radford A (1981) Transformational Syntax: A Student's Guide to Chomsky's Extended Standard Theory. New York: Cambridge University Press.

14. Sells P (1985) Lectures on Contemporary Syntactic Theories: An Introduction to Government-Binding Theory, Generalized Phrase Structure Grammar, and Lexical-Functional Grammar. Stanford, CA: CSLI/Stanford.

15. Chafe W (1994) Discourse, Consciousness, and Time. Chicago: University of Chicago Press, 17.

16. To be fair to the structuralists whom Chomsky so roundly ridiculed, it must be noted that many of them were anthropological linguists or missionaries who did go to remote areas and investigated what are to us exotic languages, such as those spoken by tribes in Africa, the peoples of the Amazon rainforests, the Australian Aborigines, and Native Americans. They did base their structural linguistics on data from these languages – and collected data on the basis of what they believed about structure. Their work has yielded highly important information about non-Aryan languages and our understanding of language in general.

17. Fromkin V (1975) A linguist looks at 'A linguist looks at "schizophrenic" language'. Brain and Language 2: 498–503.

18. Chaika E (1974) A linguist looks at 'schizophrenic' language. Brain and Language 1: 257–76.

19. Why this has been considered more scientific than simply stating that a sentence has a subject and a predicate has always been a mystery to me. What is even more of a mystery is that many brilliant scholars and students did not even realize that this is a mere restatement of an old dictum.

20. Fillmore CJ (1968) The case for case. In Bach E, Harms E (eds) Universals in Linguistic Theory. New York: Holt, Rinehart & Winston, 1–90.

21. Many linguists today would call 'Oscar' a patient as well in 'Oscar was killed.' I am an old die-hard, however, who still insists upon distinguishing between the term *object* for the thing affected when an agent or cause is stated or implied, and reserving the term *patient* for something which merely undergoes a process. My reasoning is that objects are either in direct object position after a transitive verb or, if they are in subject position, the verb is in the passive voice, whereas patients occur as subjects of intransitive verbs which can't be used in a passive construction at all. Objects must be used with transitive verbs. Patients are used as subjects of intransitives. Since objects and patients behave differently syntactically and appear in different kinds of grammatical structures, I prefer to keep them separate, but many linguists do not.

22. This book cannot digress to list fully and explain the different roles that subjects can take, but, briefly, besides being agents, causes and patients, subjects can fulfil the roles of instrumentals, locations, times, datives, beneficiaries and range (distance to destination.) Examples are, in order of mention, 'The knife cut the meat easily,' 'New York is my favourite city', 'Mornings are not my best times', 'Mary was given a promotion', 'Jack was poured coffee already' and 'Home was reached in one hour.'

23. Billow R et al. (1987) Metaphoric communication and miscomunication in schizophrenic and borderline states. In Haskell RE (ed) Cognition and Symbolic Structures: The Psychology of Metaphoric Transformation. Norwood, NJ: Ablex, 143.

24. Ruwet N (1991) Syntax and Human Experience, ed and transl Goldsmith J. Chicago: University of Chicago Press; Heine B, Claudi U, Hünnemeyer F (1991) Grammaticalization: A Conceptual Framework. Chicago: University of Chicago Press, 123–78; Heine B (1997) Cognitive Foundations of Grammar. New York: Oxford University Press; Langacker R (1998) Conceptualization, symbolization,and grammar. In Tomasello M (ed) The New Psychology of Language: Cognitive and Functional Approaches to Language Structure. Mahwah: New Jersey: Lawrence Erlbaum Associates, 1.

25. Langacker (1998) op. cit.

26. Ibid., 8.

27. Ibid., 7.

28. Ibid.
29. Chafe W (1998) Language and the flow of thought. In Tomasello M (ed) The New Psychology of Language: Cognitive and Functional Approaches to Language Structure. Mahwah: New Jersey: Lawrence Erlbaum Associates, 93–111.
30. Miller J (1995) Does spoken language have sentences? In Palmer FR (ed) Grammar and Meaning: Essays in Honour of Sir John Lyons. New York: Cambridge University Press, 116–35. Chafe W (1968) Idiomaticity as an anomaly in the Chomskyan paradigm. Foundations of Language 4: 109–27; Chafe W (1998) Language and the flow of thought. In Tomasello M (ed) The New Psychology of Language: Cognitive and Functional Approaches to Language Structure. Mahwah: New Jersey: Lawrence Erlbaum Associates, 93–111; Hanks WF (1996) Language and Communicative Practices. Boulder, Colorado: Westview Press, 61.
31. Halliday MAK (1985) An Introduction to Functional Grammar. Baltimore: Edward Arnold, 38–67.
32. Chafe W (1994) Discourse, Consciousness, and Time. Chicago: University of Chicago Press, 140–5.
33. Miller J (1995) Does spoken language have sentences? In Palmer FR (ed) Grammar and Meaning: Essays in Honour of Sir John Lyons. New York: Cambridge University Press, 116–35.
34. Chafe W (1994) Discourse, Consciousness, and Time. Chicago: University of Chicago Press, 144.
35. Ibid., 57; Johnstone B (1996) The Linguistic Individual: Self-Expression in Language and Linguistics. New York: Oxford University Press, 35.
36. Johnstone (1996) op. cit.
37. Chafe W (1994) Discourse, Consciousness, and Time. Chicago: University of Chicago Press, 139.
38. Ibid., 79.
39. Ibid., 54–6.
40. Ibid., 54.
41. Baars W (1988) A Cognitive Theory of Consciousness. Cambridge: Cambridge University Press.
42. Reason J (1984) Lapses of attention in everyday life. In Parasuraman R, Davies DR (eds) Varieties of Attention. New York: Academic Press.
43. Gazzaniga M (1992) Nature's Mind: The Biological Roots of Thinking, Emotions, Sexuality, Language, and Intelligence. New York: Basic Books; Chaika E (1995) On analysing schizophrenic speech: what model should we use?' In Sims A (ed) Speech and Language Disorders in Psychiatry. London: Gaskell, 47–56; Morice R (1995) Language impairments and executive dysfunction in schizophrenia. In Sims A (ed) Speech and Language Disorders in Psychiatry. London: Gaskell.
44. Chaika E, Alexander P (1986) The ice cream stories: a study in normal

and psychotic narrations. Discourse Processes 9, 305–28.

45. Chaika E (1990) Understanding Psychotic Speech: Beyond Freud and Chomsky. Springfield, Illinois: Charles C Thomas, 190.

46. Ibid., 206.

47. Chaika E (1982) A unified explanation for the diverse structural deviations reported for adult schizophrenics with disrupted speech. Journal of Communication Disorders 15: 167–89.

48. Chaika E (1982) Thought disorder or speech disorder in schizophrenia?' Schizophrenia Bulletin 8, 587–91; Chaika E (1990) Understanding Psychotic Speech: Beyond Freud and Chomsky. Springfield, Illinois: Charles C Thomas, 50–72.

49. Ruwet N (1991) Syntax and Human Experience, ed and transl Goldsmith J. Chicago: University of Chicago Press; Heine B (1997) Cognitive Foundations of Grammar. New York: Oxford University Press.

50. Turner M (1996) The Literary Mind: The Origins of Thought and Language. New York: Oxford University Press.

51. Chaika E (1994) Language: The Social Mirror, 3rd edn. Boston, Mass.: Heinle & Heinle; Johnstone B (1996) The Linguistic Individual: Self-Expression in Language and Linguistics. New York: Oxford University Press.

52. Chafe W (1994) Discourse, Consciousness, and Time. Chicago: University of Chicago Press.

53. Linde C (1993) Life Stories: The Creation of Coherence. New York: Oxford University Press.

54. Chafe W (1994) Discourse, Consciousness, and Time. Chicago: University of Chicago Press, 38.

55. Sacks H (1972) An initial investigation of the usability of conversational data for doing sociology. In Sudnow D (ed) Studies in Social Interaction. New York: Free Press.

56. English has a large class of two-part verbs composed of a main verb + particle. This particle is also a preposition in other usages. Two other examples of two-part verbs are *rip off* to mean 'steal,' *put out* to mean 'extinguish, as in 'put out the lights'. Francis WN (1954) The Structure of American English. New York: Ronald Press, 265–8.

57. Hanks WF (1996) Language and Communicative Practices. Boulder, Colorado: Westview Press.

58. Capps L, Ochs E (1995) Constructing Panic: The Discourse of Agoraphobia. Cambridge, Mass.: Harvard University Press; Hanks WF (1996) Language and Communicative Practices. Boulder, Colorado: Westview Press.

59. It is interesting to note that all the while Chomsky and his cohorts were actively seeking to denote their context-free generative grammars, they also made their pronouncements by saying 'In *my* dialect, I can say....', tacitly affirming that each person has his or her

own idiolect. The fact that this practice flew in the face of a notion of a grammar which generated all and only the sentences of a given language never seemed to occur to them. There can be no one set of rules to generate a grammar if individuals have rules others don't even though each recognizes that the same language is being spoken.

60. Johnstone B (1996) The Linguistic Individual: Self-Expression in Language and Linguistics. New York: Oxford University Press.
61. Quirk R, Svartvik J (1966) Investigating Linguistic Acceptability, The Hague: Mouton.
62. Johnstone B (1996) The Linguistic Individual: Self-Expression in Language and Linguistics. New York: Oxford University Press.
63. Hanks WF (1996) Language and Communicative Practices. Boulder, Colorado: Westview Press.
64. Of course, some linguists have tried to call this variation by another name, *pragmatics*.
65. Hanks (1996) op. cit.
66. Beck B (1987) Metaphors, cognition, and artificial intelligence. In Haskell RE (1987) Cognition and Symbolic Structures: The Psychology of Metaphoric Transformation. Norwood, New Jersey: Ablex, 24.
67. Ibid., 24–5.
68. Johnstone B (1996) The Linguistic Individual: Self-Expression in Language and Linguistics. New York: Oxford University Press.
69. Hanks WF (1996) Language and Communicative Practices. Boulder, Colorado: Westview Press, 93.
70. Chaika E (1977) Schizophrenic speech, slips of the tongue, and jargonaphasia: a reply to Fromkin and to Lecours and Vaniers-Clement. Brain and Language 4: 464–75; Chaika E (1982) A unified explanation for the diverse structural deviations reported for adult schizophrenics with disrupted speech. Journal of Communication Disorders 15: 167–89; Chaika E (1990) Understanding Psychotic Speech: Beyond Freud and Chomsky. Springfield, Illinois: Charles C Thomas.
71. Docherty N, DeRosa M, Andreasen NC (1996) Communication disturbances in schizophrenia and mania. Archives of General Psychiatry 53: 358–64.
72. Quirk R, Svartvik J (1966) Investigating Linguistic Acceptability, The Hague: Mouton.
73. Lorenz M (1961) Problems posed by schizophrenic language. Archives of General Psychiatry 4: 603–10.
74. Chaika E (1995) On analysing schizophrenic speech: what model should we use? In Sims A (ed) Speech and Language Disorders in Psychiatry. London: Gaskell, 55; Chaika E (1990) Understanding Psychotic Speech: Beyond Freud and Chomsky. Springfield, Illinois: Charles C Thomas, 3–49.

75. Hanks WF (1996) Language and Communicative Practices. Boulder, Colorado: Westview Press, 179.
76. Kuno S (1987) Functional Syntax: Anaphora, Discourse, and Empathy. Chicago: University of Chicago Press, 203–67.
77. Ibid., 204.
78. Ibid., 205.
79. Svartvik J (1966) On Voice in the English Verb. The Hague: Mouton, 133.
80. Chimombo M, Roseberry R (1998) The Power of Discourse: An Introduction to Discourse Analysis. Mahwah, New Jersey: Lawrence Erlbaum Associates, 108.
81. Haiman J (1998) Talk is Cheap: Sarcasm, Alienation, and the Evolution of Language. New York: Oxford University Press.
82. Ibid., 60–79.
83. Ibid., 74.

Chapter 2
Pragmatics

By considering grammar and discourse – story structure as well as story content – therapists and researchers gain access into clients' sense of themselves and others.[1]

Introduction

This chapter discusses Austin's famous lectures on how we do things with words, and Searle's Maxims of Conversation, the assumptions that help determine how we understand certain statements. The social preconditions and presuppositions that underly our speech acts are discussed. Cultural differences in practices like asking questions, interrupting others' speech, and in speaking directly are discussed. Speech act theory is applied to three therapeutic situations, showing how misunderstandings and manipulations can be effected. The role of habitual encodings in words in contributing to cultural and individual world views is also discussed, as is their importance in the therapeutic setting.

Speech acts

Austin[2] famously pointed out that a good deal of language was a way of doing things with words like betting, commanding, promising, guaranteeing, ordering (as food or services), demanding, or warning. A full discussion of speech acts,[3] as such uses of language came to be known, is beyond the scope of this book, although I have written on them extensively elsewhere,[4] and the literature on them is vast. One very important understanding that has come out of speech act theory is the degree to which we derive meaning, not just from the words and grammar that are used, but by our recognition that those words constitute a speech act. Speech acts, in and of themselves, can be created only if certain conditions are true, and part of their meaning lies in those conditions which are **preconditions** and **presuppositions**. Different speech acts have different conditions underlying them. Grice's Maxims of Conversation[5] illustrate the presuppositions underlying some speech acts.

The Maxim of Quality
Say what you believe to be true
Do not say anything for which you lack adequate evidence

The Maxim of Quantity
Do not say more than is required
Be as informative as is required

The Maxim of Relevance
Say only what is relevant to the conversation

The Maxim of Manner
Do not be obscure
Avoid ambiguity
Be brief
Be orderly

Grice himself recognized that these maxims are often flouted, but when they are they produce *implicatures*, so that if Jack says to his boss 'I can't come to work Monday because I have some physical problems that have to be taken care of', the boss supposes Jack is telling the truth (my example, not Grice's). He is telling enough, and what he has said is relevant to his not coming to work. The boss supposes, then, that Jack is going to a doctor on Monday. In actuality, Jack may have physical problems, but he really is taking Monday off because he wants to go to the circus with his children. He utilizes the social assumptions underlying statements to imply what is not true, and, by doing so, tells a lie. Note that the lie is not in what has been said, but in what Jack presumes his boss will believe from what he has said. That is, the lie is in the flouting of the maxims.

Although this example clearly conforms to Grice's maxims, as do many other exchanges, still the maxims do not constitute a complete framework for conversation. So vast and intricate is language that it would be a wonder if such a restricted set of maxims could explain all speech. Moreover, different cultures differ widely in what they consider to be direct speech, or the degree to which they insist upon indirect speech and the social settings in which each is used. Grice's maxims apply only to direct speech which is intended to communicate facts. Hanks[6] wryly comments that Grice's maxims are 'like a British philosopher's vision of what the world should be like, if only everyone had the sense to be like him'. In truth, people often varnish the truth for their own gains without creating implicature. They say more than is necessary to make their points. They chat about irrelevancies, are far from brief, and not orderly at all. It is not for nothing that we have regular discourse markers like 'As I was saying...', 'By the way...' and 'Getting back to business...'. Conversations have a nasty habit of getting off the track, tales meander, and much talk is irrelevant chit-chat. Grice's maxims seem to be accurate descriptions of what is required in scholarly writing, and even there they are often flouted, not always to produce implicatures.

In addition, these oft cited maxims are themselves vague, thus themselves flouting the maxims of quantity and manner. How does one know when one is saying more or less than is 'required'? How does one know that one is being obscure? How does one know that one's co-conversationalist doesn't recognize an item as relevant when one thinks it is relevant? How can one foresee that an utterance will be perceived as ambiguous when, in the heat of encoding one's thoughts, one doesn't see the potential ambiguity? Once, when I was speaking of a corporation which had made *fat profits*, my co-conversant surprised me by asking what fat profits had to do with our discussion. I finally discovered that she had perceived my words as *fat prophets*.

Speaking with skill also demands understanding a good deal of what the co-conversationalist is likely to know, and that is not always possible. The onus of understanding falls as squarely on the co-conversationalist as on the teller, who must rely on the other's questions to know that he or she is providing enough information. Therefore, by its very nature, conversation does not allow such maxims. At best, the maxims are goals for certain kinds of impersonal conversations and for explaining some implicatures.[7]

More to the point is that most or at least a great deal of speech is, by definition, not governed by these maxims, nor is it supposed to be. Self-abasement in politeness routines ('Oh, it was nothing'), irony, sarcasm,[8] hyperbole to underscore a point being made, all of these, by definition, do not fit Grice's maxims. When one excitedly tells a friend about a funny or dangerous incident, many details will be included that aren't strictly necessary to recount the events that occurred, but which make the story vivid and interesting. Similarly, repetitions, which violate the maxim of quantity, may be used for emphasis, comic effect, or even anger. In addition, people routinely lie. This is not necessarily done for personal gain, but to save the speaker's face, to keep him or her from having to admit to humiliating circumstances. Also, even the most honest person can't tell someone seriously that he or she looks ugly as sin, or that the dinner just served was a monument to terrible cooking. Saving other people's faces as well as one's own is a prime goal of all interaction and underlies most speaking routines.[9]

Pragmatics

Although we recognize the fuzzy border between linguistics and pragmatics, and the interdependence between them, we can still speak of the ways that language is used pragmatically. Language that is used to inform or communicate facts can be analysed in terms of how the words and syntax used add up to the intended meaning. In pragmatics, they don't. Language used pragmatically is not always used to inform. That, of course, was Austin's brilliant insight, that speech is a way of acting as much as it is a vehicle for information. One way it is used is **phatically**, as a way of allowing people to bond socially and to maintain the social status quo. Greetings, ritual complimenting, honorific address forms, and even small talk, *shooting the breeze, chewing the fat* as the idioms put it, all fall into this category.

The speech acts that Austin spoke of are also included in pragmatics. Some of these, such as betting or warning show a fit between linguistic forms used and meaning to be derived. In betting, one may say, 'I bet you that...' or one may merely say '$500 on that.' Either would constitute a bet. Similarly, warning can be very direct. 'I warn you that you will flunk this course if you persist in missing classes.' Again, however, simply stating a known danger constitutes a warning, as in 'The bridge collapsed!' 'You've missed too many classes.' Other kinds of Austin's speech acts are not usually couched directly in words and syntax that add up to their actual meaning. In an egalitarian society, those that involve asymmetrical power relations, like commanding, frequently are not. For instance, 'Excuse me, would you mind moving your cart?' although couched as an [**apology + a yes–no**] question is not asking for a *yes* or *no* response. It is actually a command 'Move your cart!' Another example occurs if I see my house-cleaner start to put on her coat and hat and I tell her, 'The living room is a mess.' She knows that I am not just keeping her abreast of the state of the house's tidiness. The apparent informative statement has the force of a command. A direct command 'Clean the living room!' too baldly brings up the power imbalance between us, that I am the superior and she is the inferior. This is not permissible in a society as egalitarian as American society pretends to be. In most instances, even those involving a disparity in rank, we usually act as if we are all equals.[10]

For a statement like 'The living room is a mess' to work as a command, unstated presuppositions and preconditions must be correct. This is typical of language used pragmatically. In this instance, the presuppositions are that the living room has not been cleaned and the cleaner has time to clean it before her work day for me is over. The preconditions are that the hired cleaner has the duty to clean the living room and I, the hirer, have the right to tell her to. That is, I have the right to command and she has the duty to carry out my command so long as it involves the job she was hired to do.

Rather than obey the command implicit in my remark, she can reply to a presupposition and say, 'I don't have time to do that room today.' She might mitigate this by prefacing her refusal with 'I'm sorry but ...' In either event, her response negates my unstated presupposition that she does have the time. Therefore, her response acceptably means 'I can't – or won't – clean the living room today.' If she responds with a tone of voice that is haughty or angry, with or without a mitigator, it could also mean 'You're all such slobs that it took me too long to clean the rest of the house.' The presupposition underlying this is that normally she can clean the living room as well as the rest of a house this size during her usual work hours, so if she doesn't have time, it's because the other rooms were so dirty. Notice the two-way indirectness of this exchange. I don't state my command directly and she doesn't express her refusal or her criticism directly, but we both understand each other. Neither of us has lost face or been insulted.

Pragmatists describe the social uses of language especially in terms of the preconditions and presuppositions that bring about the meaning of what is said. Their analyses are strongly context-based because pragmatic utterances work only in the appropriate context, and this includes the relative social statuses of interactors and the duties ascribed to them. The difference between the orientation of linguistics and pragmatics can be seen in the following common exchange:

(1). (in grocery store)
    E: (to woman in aisle) Excuse me, but where are the tomatoes?
    W: I'm sorry. I don't work here.

A linguist isolates the question and how it is derived from an underlying proposition like 'the tomatoes are $X^{location}$'. Then to form the question, the *wh*-word for denoting unknown location, *where*, is produced and preposed to the start of the sentence and the verb *are* is inverted before the subject by the general rules of English question formation, so that we end up with 'Where are the tomatoes?' W's response is formed by the rule which makes a positive sentence negative, using *don't*. The linguist could continue by showing how and why the don't occurs, but even then W's response is clearly not an answer to what was asked.

A pragmatic analysis must take account of the linguistic rules, but is more concerned with the gap between asking where the tomatoes are and the answer 'I'm sorry. I don't work here.' The answer seems to have nothing to do with the question. In order to explain this sequence, we realize that the answer is a response to the preconditions and presuppositions that govern whether a question can be asked. The preconditions are that the asker has the right to ask and the responder has the duty to answer. One precondition is that we may ask a stranger where something is in a store only if they work there. If they do work there, then they have the duty to answer. The presupposition, then, is that the person asked does indeed work there. If so, there is a further presupposition that someone who works in a store knows where things are.

W's answer literally means 'You have categorized me wrong. I don't work here so I don't have to answer your question.' or 'I don't work here so I don't know where the tomatoes are.' That this interpretation is valid is shown by a slight variation on this exchange.

(2) E: Excuse me, but where are the tomatoes?
     W: I don't work here, but the tomatoes are in Aisle 2.

Here, W answers E's presupposition that she works there, at the same time denying the precondition that she has a duty to answer. This denial is carried in 'I don't work here' which, as we've seen means 'I don't have to answer.' In contrast, W's addition of *but* means 'I'll answer your question anyway because I happen to know the answer, so I'll tell you even though I don't have to.'

The pragmatist further notes the use of politeness forms by both E and W. 'Excuse me' both alerts W that E wishes to speak with her and makes E seem to be humble.[11] Note that W matches E's politeness by saying, 'I'm sorry,' which softens her statement of refusal to answer. We see this more clearly if we consider an unlikely counterpart to (1) and (2).

(3)   E: Where are the tomatoes?
       W: What makes you think I know?

Here, E has asked too overtly so that it is heard as a demand, and W responds with hostility. Even if E, in this instance, didn't use an overt apology before asking, she could have mitigated by using a sound like 'uhhh'. Most social routines like questioning and answering or commanding and obeying serve to lessen potential animosity and to minimize confrontation. Forms of apology, *excuse me* and *I'm sorry*, as used in (1) and (2) are known as **mitigators**.

Couching my command to the housecleaner in the form of an indirect statement is also a mitigating strategy, but a weak one. If she were an equal to me, say a roommate, I would have mitigated further by asking in a light, soft voice, 'Uhhh. Would you please, if you're not too busy, clean the living room?' The 'uhh' as a marker of hesitance is a mitigator, since it signals, 'I feel hesitant to command you since you are my social equal ...' The past tense of *would* removes the request from the present, so that the request is less direct.[12] The 'if you are not too busy' further mitigates because it suggests that the other person's personal work is more important than cleaning up the mess he or she has made.

Discourse rules that are based upon preconditions and presuppositions seem to occur in most, and probably all, cultures, as does the practice of using markers of humility and mitigators. In some languages, such as Japanese, the mitigators are overt morphemes attached to nouns and verbs, morphemes which are used for no other purpose. In English, mitigators are often brought about by selection of the verb tense as well as by using a sentence form, a **locution**, that does not match what Austin called the **illocutionary force** of the statement, such as a question having the force of a command. The use of apology and a hesitant delivery are also used in mitigating in English. In general, these operate throughout the social sphere of language, including therapeutic situations.

The therapist has to be aware that clients often feel they have no right to ask questions or to challenge the therapist's conclusions. Similarly, clients can be offended by a therapist's unwitting questions. Although therapists have more leeway than the rest of us to ask certain questions, at least in the therapeutic situation, there still may be bounds on what can be asked. What it is permissible to ask questions about varies from culture to culture. For instance, a therapist in the United States can ask, 'Are you still having sex with your husband?' if the client complains about her marriage. This is a question tabooed for the rest of us in most circumstances. However, it seems to me that the therapist can't violate the general social constraint about asking someone directly how much money he or she makes or how much he or she weighs.

Even the questions that therapists have the right to ask and clients have the knowledge and duty to answer may seem intrusive or even threatening to many clients. Therapists can soften direct questions by using mitigators, saying 'Excuse me for asking, but ...' or 'By the way, had it occurred to you ...' or the like. If questions are asked without overt mitigators, then sometimes a hesitant vocal delivery combined with a soft non-authoritarian voice will achieve the same result. Therapists can also mitigate their pronouncements or solutions to clients by saying 'I think ...' 'it seems to me that ...', 'had you ever thought of ...', and the like.[13] This is not to say that therapists should speak weakly and hesitantly, as if they are sure of nothing. They must tread the fine line between speaking too positively and overbearingly, so that clients don't feel comfortable talking with them, and sounding too unsure of themselves. If therapists do not do some mitigating, however, then they are emphasizing that they are superior and the client inferior. If some mitigators are used, then the therapist is seen to be more approachable and more genuinely concerned. Whether or not questions and personal statements have to be mitigated frequently does depend partially on the culture of the client. As we shall elaborate on shortly, some cultures allow more directness than others, and therapists have to be sensitive to such issues.

Utterance pairs

Note that when discussing responses to 'Where are the tomatoes?' one option not available was for the person questioned simply not to answer, at least in Anglo-American culture. The 'Excuse me' is a sufficient interaction opener so that the person to whom it is addressed can ignore it only if he or she is deaf or very uncivil. One reason for this is that even total strangers are required to answer certain kinds of culturally dictated questions, such as asking location or time. Clearly, industrialized Westerners require these general questioning rules because there are so many new places for modern people to go to in industrial societies, either for work or pleasure. Therefore, if we come from the area, there is a general social precondition that we must all help those who are lost. Similarly, being on time is so important to our particular culture that people have to have access to knowing the time, and that sometimes involves having to ask strangers.

Few other questions can be asked of strangers. One can't go up to someone and say, 'How many children do you have?', 'What kind of job do you have?' If one did, the stranger does not have to answer and may, with justice, simply leave as fast as possible as such questions constitute bizarre statements when uttered during an initial contact with a person one doesn't know. Even at a party, where such questions are routinely asked, other politenesses usually precede the questions, and the party itself constitutes a context in which such questions are allowed between strangers. One purpose of a party can be to make new friends. Certain societal officials have the right to ask questions others can't. For instance, a police officer can and does ask strangers, 'What's your name and where do you live?' but others cannot. Many people might assume that the questioner in this instance is a police officer only because he or she asked the question!

What may and may not be asked of strangers differs among different cultures and, for the most part, what may or may not be asked is related to cultural realities. For instance, in a highly stable farming community consisting of few members, all of whom know each other, one might ask a stranger who they are and why they have come. In contrast, the Tuareg Arabs think it rude for strangers to ask who they are. One also can't ask a man his father's name in this desert culture because it is an insult equivalent to telling an adult male that he 'with all his inches of beard, is nothing save by virtue of being his father's son'. Since the Tuaregs are also nomads, and highly dependent on oases, it is considered rude to ask any question which might seem to have the intent of revealing the location of their oases. Although we are not likely to be dealing with the Tuareg, we do have to deal with people of other cultures and the therapist, especially, should be sensitive to culturally proscribed questions, or questions which might mean something different from what they do in our own cultures. Tourists in Western societies when visiting other countries do get asked by strangers where they come from. In England, it is not unusual for an American to be asked by a complete stranger, 'Do you come from America or Canada?' or 'What part of America are you from?' In America such a question does not usually get asked unless a conversation has already been initiated and the American notices the accent of the other. Even so, when Americans ask where someone is from, they often mitigate 'Excuse me, but do you come from ...?' or the like.

Questions in both European and American Anglo-based cultures[14] are part of a class of utterances which demand an appropriate response. The hearer must answer them and he or she is restricted in the forms employed when answering them. These are known as **utterance pairs**.[15] They are speech acts, if only because they force the hearer to respond. The mere utterance of the first part of such a pair acts as a command to the hearer to respond in kind, and no other material may be uttered until the utterance pair sequence is completed. These usually occur in culturally well-defined **speech events**. For instance, one greets when initiating an interaction. One complains during the speech event of the therapeutic situation, but one is not likely to complain during the speech event of a sermon in church or synagogue (although one may complain after that speech event is over). The following discussion of them does not even pretend to be complete. Only the ones most pertinent to therapy – questions and complaints – are discussed here, as well as some illustrations of how recognition of them may help in therapy.

Utterance pairs include

greeting–greeting
question–answer
complaint–commiseration, excuse, apology, or denial
request/command–acceptance or rejection (often accompanied by apology)
compliment–acknowledgement invitation
acceptance/rejection
farewell–farewell

When the first part of the utterance pair is perceived, then the proper response is made. A greeting, for instance, requires one in return. A question requires an answer and this answer must fit the form of the question. That is, a *yes*, *no*, or *I don't know* must be used to answer a **yes–no** question, and a word to fill in *when*, *why*, *where*, *what*, *which*, or *how* must be in the answer to a **wh-** question.

Greeting is important in starting any interaction, even a therapeutic one. Clients may be very put off by the therapist who fails to look them in the eye and manage a happy sounding 'Hello'. No greeting, or a lackluster one with no eye contact, indicates to clients that the therapist is bored with or even actively dislikes them. In the body of the therapeutic interview, therapists are most concerned with **question–answer** and **complaint–commiseration, excuse, apology,** or **denial**. **Excuse, apology** and **denial** usually obtain only when the complainer directly utters the complaint in face-to-face interaction with the person who caused the complaint or to one associated with that person. In terms of therapy with a third party, then commiseration is the proper second half of the utterance pair.

Since complaints, like other utterance pairs, are not overtly labelled as such, it is possible for a therapist to fail to hear a statement as a complaint. Alternatively, if the therapist does, he or she may fail to commiserate. This can be effected simply by silence. That alone can make the client feel as if the therapist doesn't care, but, as in the following interview, failure to recognize a complaint – or to respond to it sympathetically – proved to be almost disastrous.

The following is an account of part of a therapeutic session between a woman I call Helena and Dr X.Y. Here I shall concentrate on the therapist's contribution. I did attempt to contact him several times about this interchange, but was unable to contact him. In a later chapter, we shall concentrate on Helena's tale.

(4). Helena: All the time my brother and I were in school – high school and college – he made me type his papers for him. Even if it was the middle of the night, and I was asleep, I had to get up and type his papers. And his writing was so botched up that I had to literally decode what he must have meant and then put it into understandable English. It was exhausting ...

Dr X.Y. [long pause while staring at client, then sarcastically]
Ohhh, and did wé-e-e get good grades?

Helena: [no response, leaves therapist's office, recording in diary feelings of shame and inner turmoil]

This example of a therapeutic session first interested me in how therapy is done and how linguists and pragmatics could illuminate the process. The exchange shows clearly that therapy is an ordinary and usual discourse situation: a dialogue within a certain context that uses the rules and conventions of language usage. Moreover, it is a **speech event**, a definable social interaction 'delineated by well-defined boundaries and well-defined sets of expected behaviors within those boundaries'.[16] When Helena spoke, she expected the therapist to respond within those boundaries, that is, to be supportive, to ask questions about why her brother could wake her, or questions about the general family situation and Helena's role in it. She did not expect the sarcasm. A close analysis of this exchange also shows the intricate skills a speaker draws upon in even ordinary speech. Dr X.Y.'s response, far from being clumsy or obtuse shows him to be a highly skilful user of English. Why he chose to use his skill to assault his client verbally is ultimately a mystery to me, although, as noted above, I can make a conjecture,[17] but knowing the reason still wouldn't change the analysis of this extract.

The sarcasm is linguistically effected because it uses a part of our linguistic system, the pronoun *we*, and further uses vocabulary from the English speaker's stock of available words. It also uses the correct grammar rules for asking a question with a past tense verb. Pragmatically, the stress on *we* combined with an elongated downward intonation on that word, 'we-e-e', made it clear that it was being used sarcastically.

The sarcasm itself helped elucidate how the *we* was meant. In English *we* can be inclusive meaning 'you and I' or it can be exclusive, meaning 'I and one or more other persons'. The sarcasm here caused the *we* to be interpreted as *you* because it specifically obviates the relationship of 'you and I'. *You* is also ambiguous, meaning either 'you alone or 'you and one or more others'. Dr X.Y.'s use of *we* forced the meaning of '*you* and another person', namely 'you and your brother'. Since Helena was talking about her brother and herself, the sarcasm of the pronoun could only mean 'you as aide and abettor and your brother'. The effect of the sarcasm is that it names the client, as well as her brother, as cheaters. The following analysis shows in detail how this meaning is derived.

Simple sarcasm is saying something, utilizing a tone of voice, that indicates 'I mean the opposite of what the forms I'm using mean'; hence, the above *we-e-e* being construable as *you*. Haiman[18] shows that sarcasm expresses hostility towards or ridicule of another speaker, and as meaning 'X is bunk.'[19] Dr X.Y.'s sarcasm does include 'X is bunk.' However, it conveyed an even more complex meaning because Helena's story obviated such a simple reversal of meaning. In addition, the doctor's response was not to the veracity of Helena's utterance. Her brother did awaken her. She did get up and type his papers. Those facts can't be 'bunk'. Nor, apparently, did the doctor think they were since he didn't address these propositions. Therefore, the therapist's comments had to have a more complex meaning.

Dr X.Y.'s tone of voice, use of *we* and mention of grades, all made it clear that he wasn't asking a simple question. Note that Helena never mentioned grades, nor did she use the word *help* in describing what she did for her brother. The physician also didn't overtly use the word *help*. That meaning is built up from the combination of 'we', implying 'joint production', and 'get good grades'. The sarcasm conveyed, 'That you were *merely* helping is bunk', so that, in context, it only could have meant 'therefore, your "helping" was cheating'. Thus the implicature is achieved that the good grades occurred because one helped the other to achieve. The therapist interpolated the matter of grades and, by so doing, controverted Helena's tale of being oppressed so that it turned into one in which she was an active and willing participant in a fraud. The therapist completely ignored the words denoting coercion 'he made me' and 'I had to'.

Dr X.Y.'s sarcasm also conformed to the fact that sarcasts, a word coined by Haiman, 'have no wish to deceive'.[20] It seems to me that one reason that sarcasm is typically so overt is that it establishes the sarcast as being superior to the recipient of the sarcasm. This is the only explanation that I can find for his sarcasm. Helena was socially and educationally equal to him, able, for instance, to evaluate medications with the same skills he did. She had already conveyed to him her equality in prior sessions, thus unwittingly perhaps leading him to put her down so he could maintain control. One is not sarcastic with equals with whom one wishes to gain rapport, nor is one sarcastic with superiors. That his remark was to be taken to be as hostile was exhibited later when Helena confronted him with it and he sloughed it off. Finally, Dr X.Y., by giving his message sarcastically, could give an insult, and still claim innocence on the basis that he didn't come right out and say what he did, that his client was a cheat. This assault on her character uses linguistic resources for a pragmatic effect.

If the doctor had any doubts about Helena's motives, there were more neutral ways of asking. The sarcasm was created linguistically by the form of the question the therapist chose. Had he used alternative forms for *yes–no* questions, the effect would have been quite different. For instance, he could have asked 'Did your brother get good grades?' or even 'He got good grades, right?' The first, depending on the tone of voice, could be construed as a simple question asking if Helena's work was up to par, or, alternatively, it could have been construed as asking if it was worth Helena's efforts, if the brother was capable of getting good grades with her help. The second question effected by the tag, '...Right?' would presuppose that the psychiatrist thought Helena was so bright that her help would automatically gain her brother good grades. In itself, this needn't be interpreted as an accusation, provided the tone of voice in which it was delivered was friendly.

If Dr X.Y. really was morally outraged by Helena's helping her brother out by editing his work, he could have simply asked why she did it. Why did she feel she had to get up in the middle of the night to do her brother's bidding? What was there about her birth family that allowed such inconsideration?

The client made a clear complaint which required both commiseration and further questioning. To the client's shock, the physician responded with a sarcastic putdown. In effect, his response was as deviant as 'yes' would be to the question 'What time is it?' A complaint, especially in a therapeutic interview, is not supposed to be responded to with an insult to the complainer. Complaints, overt and implied, suffuse most therapeutic interactions. Indeed, the core of therapy is often to deal with complaints. Commiseration is but one response to them, perhaps the one required at the outset of the presentation of the complaint.

The next move usually should be directed towards a discussion of why or how the event occurred that caused the complaint. *Why* or *how* or any other *wh*-word is a direct invitation to open many doors to the complainer's situation, past or present. In English, complaints don't have a recognizable form such as questions or commands do. Sometimes, especially in informal situations, complaints are preceded by epithets like 'darn!' or 'Oh that slob. He's done it again!' In therapy, and out, frequently, as with Helena above, the complaint is given simply by stating an event or situation. If the event or situation described is a negative one, one in which the speaker has been disadvantaged or discomfited in any way, then the therapist is justified in hearing it as a complaint. In one way or another and to one degree or another, an event or situation described as a negative experience contains a complaint. Even the war hero describing the horrors of battle is looking for commiseration of what he had to go through as well as congratulations for having done so well that he was given a medal.

One facet of utterance pairs which should be of especial interest to therapists are the preconditions and presuppositions that lie behind the utterance pairs, and how people can manipulate each other by these. In one kind, the response includes assent to the preconditions or presuppositions of the question. For instance, one can achieve both manipulation and insult by asking questions of the form *Don't tell me you___, Are you really going to___?* or *Do you really believe___?* The presupposition behind all of these is that 'only stupid people would do or believe such a thing'. Since a question must be answered, in questions like this if the respondent says 'Yes', then he or she is admitting to the presupposition behind the question: that he or she is stupid. The respondent, to save face, might answer 'No, of course I wouldn't. I only was only kidding' or the like.

If, instead, the respondent answered 'Of course I am. Aren't you?' he or she has turned the tables on the original interlocutor, saying, in effect, 'I don't think that is stupid at all and *you* must be stupid for not doing or believing the same.' Unless the one asked is quick enough and confident enough to turn the tables, the very fact that he or she was asked a question in such a demeaning way may elicit deep-seated feelings of shame. If a client recounts such a question being asked, or, more likely, says the equivalent of 'I was going to do X, but my brother made me change my mind', the therapist's questions should be directed towards how the brother effected the change in mind. Is there a pattern of covert manipulation here? It is, of course, impossible to predict every occurrence in a therapeutic situation; however, being alive to some instances of utterance pairs, for instance, helps the therapist recognize and deal with others as they crop up.

Labov and Fanshel[21] paved the way for showing us that 'The parties to a conversation appear to be understanding and reacting to these speech acts at many levels of abstraction.' They also showed 'that actions and utterances are regularly linked together in chains of exchanges ... one of the basic strategies of the therapist is to break down the common-sense view that actions are one thing and words another'.[22] Of course, this is a restatement of the meaning of **speech act** theory as started by Austin and expanded upon by Grice and Searle, among others. Labov and Fanshel showed the degree to which utterance pairs and the underlying preconditions for them can help in understanding.

They studied the therapeutic conversations of a young woman whom they called Rhoda. Even one small part of their analysis shows the depth of understanding which can be derived when one considers speech acts and their underlying presuppositions and preconditions. The situation was that Rhoda is an anorexic. She is also in a power struggle of sorts with her mother. Rhoda insists she is old enough and responsible enough for more independence. Her mother disagrees. The mother finally leaves Rhoda at home and goes to visit and help out Rhoda's sister Phyllis. Rhoda cannot cope as well as she thought, but neither can she directly ask her mother to come home because that would be an admission that the mother is correct that Rhoda is not ready for independence. When her mother fails to come home when Rhoda expects her to, she finally calls. Rhoda reports the ensuing exchange (not in original transcription form):[23]

(5) (a) ... I called her today. I said, When do you plan to come home?
     (b) So she said, 'Oh, why?'
     (c) And I said, 'Well thing are getting just a little too much [laugh] This is
          – it's just getting too hard, and...I–'
     (d) She said to me, 'Well, why don't you tell Phyllis that?

Rhoda's mother doesn't answer the question in (a). Instead, she counters with a question of her own, (b) 'Oh, why?', which means 'why are you asking that question?' Since Rhoda as a daughter has a right to ask her mother when she's coming home, the mother's counter question, known as an **insertion sequence**, is manipulative. Clearly, given the family history, if Rhoda is asking, it is most likely that she wants her mother home because she, Rhoda, can't cope. She asks in the indirect fashion of (a), asking *when* the mother is coming, rather than directly asking her to come home. This indirection is an attempt by Rhoda to save herself the embarrassment of having to admit that her mother has been right. Rhoda isn't ready for more independence. The mother cleverly foils Rhoda so that she has to admit she can't cope in (c). Notice how much Rhoda downplays the situation. She says '*Well*, things are getting just a *little too much*! [laugh] and 'it's *just* getting too hard.' In this instance, *well* is a mitigator. It indicates that the complaint which is to follow is more trivial than it actually is. Rhoda continues with this trivialization by saying things are a *little too much* and also by using the word *just*. At this point, the mother interrupts Rhoda and delivers the *coup de grace* in (d), 'Why don't you tell Phyllis that?'

The mother very cleverly gets Rhoda to admit she can't be independent. First, she doesn't answer Rhoda's first question, which forces Rhoda to be more direct in asking her to come home. Despite Rhoda's attempt to mitigate the severity of the situation, the implication is clear that she cannot cope. Rhoda is in a classic double-bind situation. She has to ask for help, but if she does, then she will have lost the original battle with her mother. Her embarrassment in having to admit that she can't cope shows in the hesitations and false starts of (c).

The reason that I called the mother's response in (d) a *coup de grace* is that both she and Rhoda know that it is really up to the mother when she will come home. There is no precondition that says that a mother must remain in another daughter's home. In fact, the opposite is true, the mother has a prior obligation to her own household. Telling Rhoda, then, to tell Phyllis is a way of saying that Phyllis is the more important daughter, more important than Rhoda, indeed, so important that the mother is justified in neglecting her duties to her own household. Also, for Phyllis's sake, she will suppress her rights as a mother and allow Phyllis to make the decision. As Labov and Fanshel concluded, it is clear that Rhoda has been outmanoeuvred. Not only has the mother forced Rhoda into admitting she can't be as independent as she thinks, the mother has, in effect, also refused Rhoda's implicit request for help. It seems to me that this mother has also conveyed very cleverly that Phyllis is the preferred daughter and has said it so covertly that the topic can't be discussed openly.

Notice that all of this works because both Rhoda and her mother know the rights and obligations of questioners and answerers, as well as the social responsibilities of mothers and daughters to each other. The interpretation of the exact words that Rhoda and her mother used is derived from our knowledge of speech acts and how they are used in ordinary conversations. Rhoda's mother clearly knew what she was doing with her innocent sounding words and Rhoda also did. If we do not take into account the social preconditions for asking questions, the presuppositions of the interactors, and the intentions of the speakers, then Rhoda's mother's question in (b) and statement in (d) would make no sense.

Wayne Beach[24] makes a good case for studying naturally occurring social interaction in order to explain such matters as bulimia. He demonstrates that many researchers base their findings on questionnaires on the basis of which one gets the 'individual's reconstruction of social events and relationships'. Such practice leads to categorical descriptions that 'emerge from researcher imposed constructions of removed events'. That is, one can't uncover from such studies the kinds of interactions that produce specific behaviours. For that, one must study the interactions themselves. I agree. Also, any research into any social activity that relies on the subjects' memories is unreliable. First of all, different people involved in the interaction are likely to interpret their and others' roles quite differently, and, as is well-known, two people who live through the same events may each remember very different things about that event. Each may have focused on different aspects of the event; therefore, storing different versions of it. Second, as Haiman's study of alienation[25] shows, once people have left the situation, they become alienated from it, so that their descriptions of their emotions at a prior time are not necessarily what they feel now.

Beach investigated how the topic of bulimia was raised and acted upon by carefully analysing the conversation of a bulimic and her grandmother. A major issue in solving problems is raising topics and getting them discussed. Utterance pairs, because they both allow and even force a response can be employed to raise topics in an innovative manner, as we saw above. Question and answer come directly to mind, as in Rhoda's case. Other utterance pairs can also be manipulated to open up a topic.

Beach shows how a grandmother, G, tries to get her granddaughter, S, to admit she is bulimic. S both denies this and tries to avoid any discussion of it, but G is a registered nurse and sees the damage bulimia can inflict. She waits until a ripe moment to raise the topic. It comes when S gives her an invitation to take a walk together. This is the first part of an utterance pair, and calls for an acceptance or rejection. Instead, G seizes upon it as a way to raise the topic. G neither accepts nor rejects the invitation by S to go for a walk with her. This does violate the rule of utterance pairs concerning invitations, but the violation allows G to use the invitation as an entrée to the subject which bothers her, by saying 'A walk? My goodness. You're on your feet eight hours a day. You don't even have a place to sit down. Whadda you wanna go for a walk? ... that's like the postman goin' for a walk on his day off?' S explains why she likes to walk even if she is on her feet all day, and reissues her invitation. At the second instance of the invitation, G still neither refuses nor accepts, but finally says 'Well, honey, you're so thin now.' Thus the subject of bulimia is finally overtly raised. One mustn't suppose that the discussion has clear sailing from then on. It doesn't. There's a good deal of what Beach calls 'avoidance and pursuit' of the topic, but it proceeds until S admits her behaviour,[26] saying 'I got plenty of friends that do [eat, then go into the bathroom and throw up] ... How do you think I learned it Gramma?' Such an admission is a requirement before the problem can be worked out. We can credit G's controverting of the utterance pair of invitation and her persistence in the face of denial. Again, we see the value of close listening and sensitivity to the form of what is actually said. It is true that virtually all members of a society understand its utterance pairs and can manipulate them. Bringing them to the consciousness of therapists is just another way to sensitize them to the forms of speech which usually just wash right over us.

High and low involvement cultures

A major glitch in communication occurs when the therapist and the client or patient come from cultures which use different speaking styles. The early research on conversational turn-taking gave us a picture of a smooth transition between conversationalists, with conversants rarely, if ever, interrupting each other. Interruptions were seen as rudeness, even aggressiveness, as one person 'taking the floor from another'. Tannen[27] cites an article about a psychologist who considers 'fast talkers' and those who don't allow pauses between turns as being 'conversational menaces' who 'crowd' others. Notice that speaking practices are likened to actual physical behaviours. That is how vivid and forceful 'mere speech' is to people. The author of the article Tannen is quoting is speaking of individuals, but we find that there are cultures in which interrupting speakers is not only done all the time, but is felt to be a sign of caring about what the other has to say. Tannen calls these **high involvement cultures** (henceforth, HI speakers). Other **low involvement cultures** (henceforth, LI speakers) operate differently. One person doesn't speak until the co-conversant has stopped, and, typically a pause of a given length has passed. Such pauses vary with the culture. It is those of low involvement cultures who feel crowded or stepped upon by high involvement culture speakers. What Tannen's quoted author does not realize is that HI speakers feel negatively towards LI ones, because they feel that the LI speakers are remote, cold, uninterested, and difficult to talk with.

Although Tannen wrote as if we can divide all peoples as HI or LI, my own observations, living in a multicultural community and teaching college students from different ethnic backgrounds, lead me to the conclusion that there is a cline from very HI cultures to very LI ones. My own students, when asked to analyse speech at various functions, like a party, a wake, a conversation between their friends or a family dinner, have discovered that there are HI and LI social situations as well as distinct HI and LI cultures. Still, cultural differences do exist and the therapist must be aware of them. If an HI therapist is suddenly faced with a pause when it is the client's turn to speak, the therapist might jump in with more words, figuring the client didn't want to talk. However, the client, used to pausing, might just be getting ready to speak and then feels as if the carpet is being pulled from under his or her legs. As an HI speaker, I well know the discomfort of waiting for an LI speaker to take his or her part. Not speaking in my culture indicates lack of interest, disapproval or even anger. I actually feel anxious and annoyed that the other doesn't leap into his or her turn to speak. What I don't know is the discomfort of the LI speaker who feels as if he or she can never get a word in edgewise. American Southerners are considerably more LI than American Northerners. One Southern friend of mine once told me that she never got to speak at meetings or parties once she moved to the Northeast because just as she was going to say something, a Northerner butted in. In other words, the length of pause she needed before she felt she could take her turn coincided with the length of pause that the Northerner interpreted as the co-conversant having nothing to say! Also, HI speakers constantly make little comments while the co-conversant is speaking, comments like 'Oh, how awful', 'And what did you do then?', 'Tsk, you must have felt awful ...' These comments, which may be construed by some LI speakers as rude intrusions, are very encouraging to HI speakers, making them feel that the listener really cares.

In addition, HI speakers tend to use fewer mitigators and hedges than LI ones do. HI speakers state things directly 'bald on record'. Therefore, they often come across as being very sure of themselves, to the point of arrogance. Such differences between communicative styles are heightened in therapy which, after all, depends on conversational practices. To complicate matters, all clients, HI as well as LI, often speak indirectly of what they are ashamed or pained by or they avoid mention entirely. It is the therapist's job to get them to talk about what is really bothering them, and to do this the therapist has to match their conversational mode. Although even HI speakers find it difficult to speak baldly in a therapeutic situation, eliciting speech from them is more successful if the therapist makes quiet encouraging comments, such as those mentioned above. LI speakers are more likely to clam up if such comments are made while they are talking. They typically require gentler prodding and indirect questions. HI therapists must practise hedging and mitigating so as not to appear threatening and authoritarian to any of their clients, HI as well as LI. The therapist, especially an HI one, must learn to wait for the pauses between utterances the LI client needs, but LI therapists must be aware of how uncomfortable HI clients may be if such silences occur. It is up to the therapist to be aware of these cultural differences and to be prepared to adjust his or her own way of speaking accordingly. Otherwise, rapport will be difficult to achieve.

How can the therapist tell whether the client belongs to an LI or an HI culture? There is no surefire litmus test I know of except to listen to how the client talks during the first interviews. The therapist can note if the 'encouraging remarks' make the client stop speaking or react by looking away, squirming and other signs of discomfort. The therapist can also see if such remarks do encourage the client to keep on speaking. This, combined with the directness of the client's speech and whether or not the client habitually allows a lapse of silence in between responses can help the therapist identify the client's speaking style.

A good example of the contrast between speaking styles occurred while I was sitting in on a group therapy session led by Mrs Jenny France at Broadmoor Hospital in the UK. Nobody spoke until the previous speaker had not only finished but a long pause accrued. The speech therapist, Mrs. France, also let long pauses elapse before she made a comment or asked another question. To me, as an HI Northern American speaker, the pause length between turns was so uncomfortable at times I actually felt a strong urge to say something to make things right, so to speak. It took tremendous self-control just to sit quietly in my seat during the silence. Of course, I didn't say anything. I had no right to participate in the discussion at all.

After the session, I commented to the group that I was amazed that nobody broke in on anyone else, and that turntaking was so orderly. Surprisingly, the men suddenly came to life and, all talking together, excitedly asked if I had seen the *Ricky Lake Show*, an American talk show. It seems as if the guests on that show interrupt each other all the time and so intrusively that these patients found it both exciting and strange, almost incredible behaviour. While telling me about the show, it was interesting to note that more than one patient spoke at a time, they intruded upon each other's speech, and their voices were louder and more animated than during the therapy group. It was almost as if I had given them licence to talk the way people did on this show. I must stress that the therapy session, as LI as it was, was actually an excellent discussion, really getting to the bottom of how people felt and acted. Neither kind of speaking style is better than the other. Both work equally well for their speakers.

Although Tannen and I come from the same kind of HI culture, it must be emphasized that, besides the Southerners mentioned above, members of some ethnic American cultures are very LI. It is useful to note the degree of indirection speakers from such cultures employ as opposed to the bald-on-record statements of HI cultures. An ethnically French-Canadian American colleague of mine who, like me is a Northerner and even graduated from the same university as I, seemed very preoccupied at a faculty dinner one night. I asked him what the problem was. He complained angrily to me that his son and daughter-in-law always brought their new baby girl to the maternal grandparents' home every Sunday so that by the time the baby came to my colleague's home, she was cranky. I said, indignantly, 'Why don't you tell them "Hey, you should come to our house first some time so we can enjoy the baby."' 'Oh, no!,' came the shocked response. 'The next time they come over, I'll just hand the baby to them and say, "Here, she's tired now. Take her home."' It was my turn to be shocked. 'Will they understand that?' to which he replied, 'Of course.' I know if I were to speak so indirectly to my children, they would assume that I didn't want to see them or their babies. However, my colleague was right. The following Sunday the baby was brought to his house first. His son understood perfectly.

Cultural differences in communicative styles are not the only source of fumbling. Conversants may misinterpret what is in the other's mind, such as what intention the other had in saying what he or she did. Sometimes one or the other conversant is distracted, or one party assumes background knowledge or assumptions the other doesn't have. Sometimes the therapist misses the client's cues which are indirect invitations to open some line of inquiry, as in the dialogue between Dr X.Y. and Helena. Finally, we can admit that giving the right response can be a very difficult matter in a therapeutic situation. The right response depends upon the individual's personality, his or her cultural group, and the nature of his or her problem. The therapist has to be aware of cultural differences and also be very sensitive to language and to the client's responses to what is asked or said.

Habitus

The diverse ways that humans categorize their world, what Hanks[28] calls **habitus**, strongly affect the way people interact with the world. Habitus is 'the embodied inclination of agents to evaluate and act on the world in typical ways'.[29] Without thinking, so to speak, people make certain assumptions about their world and act according to those assumptions.

These assumptions are codified largely because of habitual ways of speaking about things as well as because of the ways one language codifies the world. This doesn't mean that people are prisoners of their languages. Habitus is as flexible as language itself is. So, although we may unthinkingly adopt a certain stance or assume a certain meaning in events, new experiences may change the stance or the assumption. Hanks[30] notes that all people who speak a certain language do not necessarily 'share the same routinized dispositions to perceive objects the same way or to engage in verbal practices the same way'. He believes that, like grammar, habitus is highly differentiated according to one's social status and role.

Since habitus is built upon experience, it seems to me that there are individual as well as group differences in orientation to the world. For this reason, I think that the concept of habitus is useful for therapists. Not only does it alerts therapists to expect differences in world view from members of different social groups, differences that affect individuals' behaviour, but also to expect important differences among individuals. For some persons the world is a very different place to live in than mine is, for instance. We shall see this in Chapter 6 when we discuss Clive, Meg, Nate and Esther. Meg, an agoraphobic, lives in a world where unpredictable forces can take over her body, throwing her in a panic. Clive sees the world as a series of lucky or unlucky events which cause things to happen to him, and Esther sees it as a dangerous place inhabited almost entirely by her enemies. Any new experience becomes a reinforcer of the habitus because people fit the new event into the world they've constructed. Each has a habitus which causes him or her to interpret new events in particular ways, ways perhaps most of us would never think of. This isn't to say that one can't find a group of people like Meg, Clive or Esther. Indeed, one can. That is why we have names like *agoraphobia*, *schizophrenia* and *paranoia* to describe such people, but these terms cut across social class and social roles, and the sufferers do not usually cohere into a group. Rather, they stand out as anomalies within their social group.

The diverse ways that humans categorize their world, their habitus, strongly affect the way they interact with the world. One recent, tragic example of conflict of habitus was seen in America with a confrontation between a group of families called the Branch Davidians and the US Government's Bureau of Alchohol, Tobacco, and Firearms (ATF), a confrontation ending in several deaths of the very people the ATF was supposed to be saving. The Davidians saw themselves as a religious group and the ATF saw them as a dangerous cult. The latter had been sent to break up the Davidian group and to seize their weaponry. On their part, the Branch Davidians looked upon the ATF as dangerous intruders, bent on destroying their home and their religion. When the ATF called in tanks, the Davidians looked at the awesome warlike government machinery and saw Armageddon, not law and order. The ATF looking at a 'cult' saw a bunch of dangerous misfits who had little children living with them. The government agents did not recognize that the Davidians saw themselves as beleaguered and trying to defend their home and families from the enemy which, to them at that time, was the United States government. What the ATF personnel saw both as a rescue mission to get people out of the clutches of the cult, as well as an official mission to seize illegal guns, the Davidians saw as a vicious attack. Perhaps if the government had seen the Davidians as a group of families with a *bona fide* religion, as people living according to their religious beliefs, and with the right to live that way, the ATF personnel would have handled the entire matter more tactfully. The outcome might have been quite different had a more indirect politeness prevailed rather than the overt display of power.

The concept of habitus leads us to our own stances. We say certain people 'don't listen to reason'. The very concept of listening to reason implies that the speaker is the reasonable one and is speaking from a specific habitus, the way one views and acts upon the world. Any departure from that habitus is likely to be perceived as not being reasonable. If, as in the cases of the agoraphobic, the schizophrenic or the paranoid, the habitus is dysfunctional, not allowing its sufferer to participate with joy in the world or keeping them disabled, then part of what must be strived for is to get them to change their world view. Meg has to learn that unpredictable forces don't take over her body. Clive has to learn that he plays an active role in what happens to him, and Esther, now deceased, might have been encouraged to see that every remark made to her was not intended as a putdown or expression of hostility. This doesn't mean even the best of therapists are going to succeed in effecting such changes in clients with such deeply ingrained views of the world, but if the therapist is at least aware, he or she can try to make the client more flexible in his or her understanding of the world. For instance, for those like Esther, one can ask exactly what the offending person said. Then, it can be suggested that those words have different meanings as well, and a discussion can ensue of what was said and all the things it could mean. This helps teach flexibility in interpreting others' actions and should also show that the remarks in question were not necessarily those of an enemy. Certainly, just doing this once is not sufficient, but, if it is done enough, it becomes routine practice, and routine practice is powerful in building up our imagery of the world and our interactions with it.

For many years, mainstream linguists, including me, derided or ignored the anthropologists who dared say that one's language influenced how one sees the world. This was known as the Sapir–Whorf theory. These anthropologists noted that many languages did not have the same categories, for instance, for time that European languages do. Therefore, so the theory went, the speakers of those languages didn't cut up events into little chunks of time. They saw things more fluidly. Mainstream linguists pooh-poohed such theorizing on several grounds. First, every language can change to accommodate new meanings. Second, it was argued, all languages do the same things, albeit in different ways, so, if the Navajo language, for instance, didn't use tense markers on verbs, that didn't mean the Navajo had a radically different conception of time from Anglos. Their language had other terms for time. Moreover, it seems to me that if Navajos don't – or didn't – chunk the days up into seconds and hours as obsessively as Anglos do, it was because they had no cultural reason to do so. Most industrialized people from Western cultures have had the experience of 'losing track of time' when doing enjoyable things or when on vacation, but as soon as they're back at work, then time matters and suddenly the minute hand on the watch regains its pertinence. Also, the Chinese languages do not have verb tense either, yet nobody could say their civilization doesn't pay attention to time in much the same way as Western cultures do. They simply use time words like adverbials to indicate time, rather than attaching a tense morpheme on to verbs. Even in a European language like English, tense markings don't necessarily indicate time. The so-called present tense, for instance, can be used for the future or the past as in

(6)   (a) The plane *leaves* tomorrow.
      (b) There I *am*, my keys *are* in the car, and it *is* pouring rain.

In 6(a) the notion of future is on the adverb *tomorrow*, and the verb is in present tense. The predicament in 6(b) is clearly about a past event, but it is expressed in the present tense. Capps and Ochs[31] show how an agoraphobic, whom they call Meg, feeds her fears by constant repetition of anecdotes of when she suffered panic attacks. Often when she does this, she uses the present tense as if she were undergoing the panic again while telling of it. This is one of the mechanisms Meg uses to reinforce her illness.

Hanks defends Whorf, however, very reasonably. He reminds us of **deictics**. Some languages have these encoded in their grammar. These are the words in a language which point out location, time, or things. Their meaning is wholly determined by context. Words like *there*, *here*, *this*, *that*, *now*, *soon* and *later* are all deictics. So are such things as verb tense markers. Hanks[32] asserts that if a feature of context, such as time, is encoded on to the grammar of a language, 'speakers using the language are habituated to take notice of the corresponding aspect of context'. Thus these aspects of context become powerfully routinized because of the frequency of their mention and 'provide a privileged window' on how the speakers categorize existence. In terms of time, this would mean that speakers of a language which did grammaticize time as obligatory tense markers would always be far more influenced by time than those whose language was tense-free. Although this is an empirical matter, Hanks does not cite tests which show that this is true. There is a body of testing that has been done on speakers whose languages use shape markers on nouns or whose languages cut up the colour spectrum differently from Europeans. The purpose of these tests has been to see if those who use shape markers are quicker at identifying shapes than those who speak European languages who don't use shape markers. The colour tests are to see if people are quicker to recognize colours their language names as primary than are speakers of languages which treat colour differently. Such testing has shown that the grammatical categories or colour coding does not permanently affect speakers' performances on tests.[33] How valid Hanks assertion is in terms of deictics or any other grammatical function's influencing its speakers' experience of existence, I don't know. Syntactic rules, and these include usage of such matters as tense markers, usually operate well below the level of consciousness. Moreover, as in English, typically syntactic markers for tense are used for purposes other than signalling time even if we name them as time markers by using words like *past*, *present* and *future*.[34] *Mutatis mutandis* this may be true of other syntactic categories in English and other languages.

However, we can readily see how certain habitual encodings on to lexical items or habitual language practices do influence people's attitudes and experiences of the world in other ways. The large literature that now exists on propaganda shows how lexical items influence attitudes.[35] Hanks is talking about entire language systems including our barely noticed employment of syntactic rules, but individuals use their own language habitually to encode events, and the way they do this strongly affects their thinking and their behaviours (Chapter 5).

Take the matter of utterance pairs. Our own linguistic habits for these have to be deeply ingrained in us as all of our social practices operate through them. Kinesics, body motion and eye gaze are also highly routinized behaviours in a culture and we rely upon these in categorizing and judging co-conversants. Native Americans don't feel the same constraints to respond immediately to a question that Anglos do.[36] Consequently, Native Americans have often been perceived by Anglos as passive and uninterested. This feeling is intensified because Native American eye gaze and body motion are so different from those of Anglos. The Native Americans don't look at their interlocutors as frequently or for as long as do Anglos and their bodies are less animated than Anglos are used to.[37] Anglos perceive this as further indication that Native Americans are too passive as well as uninterested in things. In turn, Native Americans view Anglos as aggressive and controlling and, of course, rude. They construe Anglo eye-contact practices as staring. Perception of peoples out of one's social group, then, is strongly affected by habituated cultural behaviours. As Hanks[38] puts it 'the vast majority of our knowledge of the social world comes not from direct experience with objects and other people but from the system of social typifications, through which we understand direct experience in terms of typical categories'. Since the Native American typifications match the dominant Anglo categories of passivity and unintcrcst, then therapists are likely to experience such behaviour in those terms. Typification can be in the language itself or in the ways a particular group carries out linguistic communication. Therapists especially have be aware of the degree to which their perceptions of clients are influenced by such typifications, especially if they are treating those of another culture. If the client appears too passive, is it because his or her eye gaze, body motions, and facial expressions are culturally different from the therapist's? Or is it because the client is truly passive? The same questions could be asked of the client who appears too aggressive or forward.

Even within social groups, habituation towards attitudes is also effected through certain language practices. Recent work, much of it on propaganda, news reporting and the like, has shown that people are highly influenced by the phrases habitually used in their culture to define or describe.[39] For instance, newspapers habitually refer to management's having labour troubles. This makes people think of labour causing problems, so that labour is at fault in disputes. If, instead, papers reported that labour has management troubles, management would be perceived as the problem, not labour. Similarly, expressions like 'the Christian thing to do' repeated frequently make it appear as if the Christian thing is not only moral and correct, but that non-Christians are not synonymous with moral goodness. Compare, for instance, if one heard the comment 'That was the Moslem thing to do' or 'That was the Jewish thing to do.' Imagine what would prompt the reference to Moslems or Jews as opposed to Christians in such an expression. Terms like 'Christian charity' have the same effect of claiming a virtue for Christians and not acknowledging that other religions have the same virtue. Indeed, Christian charity derives from Jewish charity, which is an all-encompassing feature of Jewish moral tenets, as it is, I am told, of Moslem belief.

History books used to – and perhaps still do to some extent – make remarks about 'The first white man who discovered...' Such expressions carry with them the attitude that only white men count. The experiences of non-whites do not count, thereby affirming that non-whites, especially those still in tribal cultures, are virtually subhuman. The strength of this attitude is affirmed by looking at the massacres of Aborigines in Australia and New Zealand when the civilized white man came on to the scene. More recently, newspapers reporting on the Million Man March of African-American males, used verbs like '*converged* in Washington' and '*swarmed* through the streets,' and '*clogging*' the roads. The images conveyed were first of an almost military action of parallel lines of people coming together according to plan. Then the image of swarming specifically elicited insects, and, of course, clogging is not only undesirable, but carries strong imagery of plumbing failure with rather disgusting results. Had, instead, the papers described the African-Americans as convening or simply meeting, the event would not have been seen as so ominous. To have further mentioned the obvious, that a million men were going to cause some traffic jamming was not strictly necessary, but if the newspapers felt they had to point out the obvious, then a more neutral word like *fill* could have been used. What was reported both denigrated the purpose of the march and reinforced cultural attitudes that African-American males are dangerous and, to boot, like insects or other harmful materials. People form their opinion from the way something is reported, and they do so unconsciously. The status quo is very much maintained by newspaper reporting, textbook writing, and common expressions.

In sum

This chapter has shown that speaking is not a random activity, that what we say is not a simple matter of adding up basic meanings of the words used in conversation or writing. In the cases of Helena and Rhoda, we saw that sticks and stones can break our bones and, as well, words can certainly hurt us. In a later chapter we shall see the full damage done to Helena by this exchange. Finally, we have seen the degree to which cultures may vary in their use of language and body motions, a fact of which many therapists in urban areas around the world need to keep reminding themselves.

Notes

1. Capps L, Ochs E (1995) Constructing Panic: The Discourse of Agoraphobia. Cambridge, Mass.: Harvard University Press, 178.
2. Austin JL (1975) How to Do Things with Words, 2nd edn., Urmson JO, Sbisè M (eds). Cambridge, Massachusetts: Harvard University Press.
3. Searle JR (1969) Speech Acts: An Essay in the Philosophy of Language. Cambridge: Cambridge University Press.
4. Chaika E (1990) Understanding Psychotic Speech: Beyond Freud and Chomsky. Springfield, Illinois: Charles C Thomas, 150–83.
5. Ibid., 163–5.
6. Hanks WF (1996) Language and Communicative Practices. Boulder, Colorado: Westview Press, 99.
7. Chaika E (1990) Understanding Psychotic Speech: Beyond Freud and Chomsky. Springfield, Illinois: Charles C Thomas, 163–70.
8. Haiman J (1998) Talk is Cheap: Sarcasm, Alienation, and the Evolution of Language. New York: Oxford University Press, 98–9.
9. Goffman E (1995) On face work. Psychiatry 18: 213–31.
10. Exceptions to this include special situations in which the line of command must be maintained, such as the military, police, firefighters, or surgeons in an operating room.
11. It is common in many languages for a questioner, or any interactor, to pretend to be humble. 'Excuse me' is a pretence of asking for forgiveness for intruding upon another. Only an inferior has to ask such forgiveness.

12. Some languages, like Japanese, actually have sets of suffixes to put on verbs to soften their impact. In English, this is usually done by using the past tense and modal auxiliaries like *will, would, can, could*. A similar usage is seen when a clerk in a store says to a customer, 'That will be $5.00 please.' The use of the future again makes the request less direct because it pretends not to be speaking of the here and now.

13. These suggestions are not ad hoc. They are derived from the literature on how people, especially women in our culture, lessen the impact of their statements, and on the literature of sociolinguistic studies of Japanese culture, a culture which avoids direct bald-on-record statements. It is clear from extensive studies in sociolinguistics that hedged and mitigated statements are less threatening than are direct ones. Similarly, a forceful, non-hesitant speaking style is more threatening than a soft-voiced hesitant one.

14. Many Native Americans do not share in the culturally based forced response. For instance, when asked a question, a Warm Springs Indian might not give an answer to it for days, when the time is ripe, so to speak. Philips SU (1970) Acquisition of rules for appropriate speech usage. In Alatis J (ed) Bilingualism and Language: Anthropological, Linguistic, Psychological, and Sociological Aspects, Monograph series on Languages and Linguistics. Washington, DC: Georgetown University Press; Philips SU (1976) Some sources of cultural variability in the regulation of talk. Language in Society 5: 81–95.

15. Chaika E (1994) Language: The Social Mirror, 3rd edn. Boston, Mass.: Heinle & Heinle, 173–93; Sacks H (1992) Lectures on Conversation, Vol. 1, Jefferson G (ed). Cambridge, Mass.: Blackwell.

16. Labov W, Fanshel D (1977) Therapeutic Discourse. New York: Academic Press, 30.

17. I did try to contact the therapist several times asking him if he had any special therapeutic purpose in mind or if he could explain things differently. However, he did not answer my letters about this interaction or any others cited in this book. He did know how I was interpreting them.

18. Haiman J (1998) Talk is Cheap: Sarcasm, Alienation, and the Evolution of Language. New York: Oxford University Press, 25.

19. Ibid., 21.

20. Ibid.

21. Labov W, Fanshel D (1977) Therapeutic Discourse. New York: Academic Press, 364.

22. Ibid., 29–30.

23. Ibid., 364.

24. Beach WA (1996) Conversations about Illness: Family Preoccupations with Bulimia. Mahwah, New Jersey: Lawrence Erlbaum Associates, 102–12.

25. Haiman J (1998) Talk is Cheap: Sarcasm, Alienation, and the Evolution of Language. New York: Oxford University Press.
26. Beach WA (1996) Conversations about Illness: Family Preoccupations with Bulimia. Mahwah, New Jersey: Lawrence Erlbaum Associates, 72.
27. Tannen D (1984) Conversational Style. Norwood, N.J.: Ablex, 78.
28. Hanks WF (1996) Language and Communicative Practices. Boulder, Colorado: Westview Press, 237–41.
29. Ibid., 239.
30. Ibid.
31. Capps L, Ochs E (1995) Constructing Panic: The Discourse of Agoraphobia. Cambridge, Mass.: Harvard University Press.
32. Hanks WF (1996) Language and Communicative Practices. Boulder, Colorado: Westview Press, 179.
33. Kay P, Kempton E (1984) What is the Sapir–Whorf Hypothesis? American Anthropologist 86: 65–79.
34. Lakoff R (1972) Language in context. Language 48: 907–27; Quirk R, Greenbaum S (1973) A Concise Grammar of Contemporary English. New York: Harcourt Brace Jovanovich, 40–58.
35. van Dijk T (1988) News as Discourse. Hillsdale, NJ: Lawrence Erlbaum; Macedo D (1994) Literacies of Power: What Americans Are Not Allowed to Know. Boulder: Westview Press.
36. Philips SU (1970) Acquisition of rules for appropriate speech usage. In Alatis J (ed) Bilingualism and Language: Anthropological, Linguistic, Psychological, and Sociological Aspects, Monograph series on Languages and Linguistics.Washington, DC: Georgetown University Press.
37. Chaika E (1994) Language: The Social Mirror, 3rd edn. Boston, Mass.: Heinle & Heinle, 144–5.
38. Hanks WF (1996) Language and Communicative Practices. Boulder, Colorado: Westview Press, 129.
39. van Dijk T (1988) News as Discourse. Hillsdale, NJ: Lawrence Erlbaum; Fairclough N (1989) Language and Power. Language in Social Life Series. New York: Longman; Macedo D (1994) Literacies of Power: What Americans Are Not Allowed to Know. Boulder: Westview Press.

Chapter 3
Doing therapy

Narrative translates knowing into telling; of fashioning human experience into structures of meaning.[1]

Introduction

This chapter discusses therapy as a way of teaching clients to talk freely and without shame, showing that therapy is a speech event jointly produced by client and therapist. It stresses the importance of not presuming what a client must feel or why, enlarging on the story of Helena introduced in the last chapter. The causes of depression are discussed in depth. Sociolinguistic concepts like face-saving, formality vs solidarity, and the achievement of rhapsody in conversation are presented.

Ego and social behaviours

Therapy is not an isolated activity. Ordinary speech behaviours conform to the very same conditions that occur in therapeutic situations. All our speaking practices gibe, in or out of therapy. The very accents we adopt, for instance, are closely related to the image we wish to present to others. So does the grammar we choose. The person who wants to be thought of as tough and macho will speak differently, such as using non-standard forms like double negatives, from the one who wishes to be thought of as educated and wise and who, consequently uses erudite words even when inappropriate socially. Labov[2] found that high-school students living on Martha's Vineyard who wanted to remain on the island after graduation, used an exaggerated Vineyard accent, but that those who chose to leave for better job opportunities spoke like Bostonians. The Vineyard accent also correlated with how strongly an individual felt that the island belonged to his or her family, and not to the interloping tourists. What this and subsequent studies of other communities showed is that people reveal their attitudes, including their sense of affiliation, and their feelings about themselves by the speech forms they adopt.

A client's speech may be filled with weak and tentative language, filled with hedgings like 'I may be wrong but ...' or 'If you really wouldn't mind ...' This portrays a portrait of a helpless, weak person casting herself or himself on the hearer's mercy. In contrast is the person who makes unvarnished pronouncements about all topics, who may even preface remarks with expressions like 'Don't tell me ...' This person wants to be seen as strong, not needing help, and knowing everything. This doesn't mean that the speaker *is* strong and doesn't need help. It may well simply signal that the speaker actually has a very poor self-image, so poor that he or she has to pretend invulnerability for fear that others will judge him or her as being weak. It's a form of hiding-out in plain view. Such people feel so inferior that they feel their 'face', their self-worth, is constantly under attack, so that the bragging and pronouncements are a form of protection. They are trying to defend themselves against humiliation. Now, this is not a new idea in therapy. The idea of an inferiority complex being the cause of egotism comes from the early days of psychotherapy. In fact, it is virtually an old saw that the person who brags a lot, who always makes stentorian pronouncements, is one who really feels inferior. We certainly have to consider that a know-it-all or obnoxious braggart might be hiding an inferiority complex, but it is also true that he or she might not be.

So far as I know, neither Freud nor Jung, nor any of their followers, nor anyone at all, has presented formal studies confirming that inappropriately superior behaviour always masks feelings of inferiority. Such studies would be demanding and take years to complete, but not necessarily impossible. It may well be that some people truly feel superior even to their peers or their therapists. Indeed, most of us feel truly superior in one way or another to some members of society. Therapists, to be credible, have to be seen as being more insightful than their clients or patients. The braggart, the know-it-all, the one with aristocratic manners may seem to present special problems in therapeutic situations, as they are less likely to heed their therapists than are less positive people.

Actually, for the therapist, the question is moot. Either way, whether the client seems weak or strong, the therapist is safer matching the degree of formality set by the client. The one who presents hesitancy and shyness will respond best to quiet, gentle tones, perhaps to mutual first-naming. Most of us can handle people easily if they act as if they are inferior to us. We try to make them at ease, and we suppose that they will listen to our pronouncements and act upon them with no questioning.

The rigid know-it-all presents more of a problem for most therapists. One can assume that if the client has come to the therapeutic situation voluntarily, he or she realizes the need for help. However, helplessness doesn't come easy to some people. By matching a superior style with formality, the therapist allows such a client to save face and still receive help. The therapist must remain sensitive to the possibility that such a client will easily find a direct comment too probing or too critical. With such clients, the therapist must employ the hedges, 'It seems to me that ...'. 'Perhaps, ...' at least until the client relaxes. There is good sociolinguistic research that reveals that it is entirely appropriate to match one's style to one's co-conversant. Style is a kind of command to the hearer that the speaker wishes to be treated with a certain amount of formality or intimacy, and it is natural in most interaction to match style with style.[3] The client may well take a therapist's attempt to be friendly and, for instance, to use first-names as a way of undermining the respect with which the client wishes to be treated. Similarly, the therapist who interrupts such a client, asks searching questions, or makes pithy comments can be inviting aloofness or even anger at best. At worst, the client won't return for the help he or she may very badly need.

What we have to remember is that this doesn't mean that all people who act as if they are superior beings have inferiority complexes. Some people seem truly to feel superior to others, even those who are ostensibly their peers. Others – manics, for instance – may be going through a phase of megalomania in which they make grand claims for themselves and who they are. Some schools of psychiatry claim that an overwhelming feeling of inferiority is a cause of mania. It is a defence mechanism, another originally psychiatric term that has passed into general vocabulary. Whether or not this is so, I don't know. There are no controlled studies of manics or even of normals who behave like know-it-alls that show such people are, indeed, suffering from feelings of inferiority which they are desperately trying to hide. Those suffering from mania might be victims of a neurochemical imbalance or they might be suffering from extreme feelings of inferiority, or both. I certainly don't know which and I've studied conversations with normal and mentally ill people for almost three decades. Although it sounds callous, it seems to me that it makes no difference whether obnoxious know-it-alls or manics have overwhelming underlying feelings of inferiority. The therapist must be prepared to adjust his or her style to that most appropriate to a given client. The know-it-all may be irritating and obnoxious for most therapists to deal with, but that doesn't mean that such people can't be borne and can't benefit from therapy. The therapist just has to recognize that he or she can't always be the one overtly in-the-know. Typically, the person with higher status has the right to determine the degree of formality that a speech event will be conducted in.[4] The therapist may not always have that luxury, but, by giving it up with some clients, the therapist has a chance of getting through to them, eventually gaining their trust and respect.

Therapy as teaching

Sue

While doing research at Broadmoor Hospital in Crowthorne, Berkshire, UK, I was privileged to be hosted by a speech therapist, Mrs Jenny France. With the patients' permission, Mrs France allowed me to sit in on several therapeutic sessions. The first was Sue, whose story was sad, but whose future was perhaps not without hope. Sue's case history is dismal. She had been abandoned by her mother at age 11 and left with her alchoholic father. She had been raped repeatedly by many men, and admitted that she had 'gone with' others casually. Not surprisingly, she used drugs and sniffed fumes. The latter, especially, seemed to have caused organic damage. Although formal IQ tests measured her only at 70, she did write poetry spontaneously. Jenny France's job, of course, was to help Sue feel better about herself so that she could eventually be released at least to a half-way house. To this end, Mrs. France had asked Sue to make a list of words about herself, which she did. She applied the following to herself: *slag, dog, easy, guilt, shame, revenge, afraid, confused*. Jenny France insightfully pointed out to me the link between Sue's negative words about herself, calling herself slag, a dog, and easy, and the other words on the list. *Guilt* and *shame* show that Sue is aware of society's evaluation of females who indulge in casual sex, but the next word, *revenge*, shows that Sue realizes she's been exploited, even though she does blame herself for being used sexually. The last two words, *confused* and *afraid* speak for themselves.

The speech therapist's aim is to give the patient a different set of words to describe herself, to develop choices in her vocabulary. To that end, Mrs. France had given Sue a notebook to keep a diary. In this, in each session, Sue underlines all the good things she has done. All of her accomplishments are written down, including such matters as her attempts to joke with others, her general friendliness, the little kindnesses she does each day. This notebook also allows Sue to keep a record of her successes in daily activities. From this notebook, Sue will build up a different set of descriptive words about herself and, eventually, a life story that includes self-respect. Mrs France told me that having Sue describe herself in good terms increases her vocabulary about herself and gives her more choices in building up her ego.

Julia

Mrs. France is exceptionally sensitive to the power of language and she uses that sensitivity skilfully in teaching or reteaching patients how to use it. She adapts her methods according to the individual. Sue was very outgoing and talkative and very amenable to keeping a diary. Julia, in contrast, spoke little and made little eye contact. She evinced a distinct paucity of verbal output. Julia had been diagnosed as schizophrenic, but, at the time I observed, she was not exhibiting symptoms such as hallucinating, expressing delusions or engaging in bizarre behaviours. She had a flat affect and made no attempt to be friendly or even likeable. This is to be expected in schizophrenics with negative symptoms.

Mrs France was trying to teach Julia basic conversational skills. To that end, Mrs France used very concrete conversational practices, for example asking Julia about the here and now, such as 'What did you do today?', 'What did you do this week?', 'What did you buy in the canteen?', 'Do you go to the discos?' Julia's answers were curt and often vague, so Mrs France then asked more questions, questions specifically based upon Julia's responses, in order to teach Julia to include more information in her answers. She thereby got Julia to elaborate. This sort of concrete here and now language learning is how children learn language and social routines.

At the same time as trying to improve Julia's conversational skills, Mrs France was working with her to retrieve earlier memories, going from questions about the present to those about the past. Although Julia claimed to remember nothing, when Mrs France asked her if she had ever had a birthday party as a child, Julia did remember having one party when she was 9 or 10. The therapist's approach here is an entry into earlier experiences by teaching the patient to elaborate on her answers about the present and to give the patient some sense of what a sufficient answer is. This is done by getting her to enlarge on her sparse responses by the therapist's asking very specific questions about them, but without pushing or repeating the questions. If the therapist were to repeat her questions, it would sound demanding or insistent and this would negate what she is trying to teach the patient. In other words, through using normal conversational techniques, the patient is being taught to articulate experiences.

The reason for trying to access earlier experiences is that if a life story can be retold (in the sense of changing the old one), then the life can be changed (Chapter 6). Obviously, a patient like Julia will need a long period of conversational therapy before she is ready to talk in any depth about her earlier years.

Being privileged to observe Mrs France's tough cases at a later stage of development, I see the possibility of hope for Julia. These tough cases were in an all male group therapy session.

The group

In her leadership of a group therapy session, Jenny France again demonstrated her understanding of the power of language change in getting people to change their self-image, to broaden their horizons of self-expectation and, mostly, because the men in this group had histories of violence, in teaching them non-violent solutions to events. As with her work with individuals, Mrs France taught social interactive skills to the group by direct questioning. Each group member took his turn in response to her questions of what had been going on in his life since the last session, how he was feeling, who visited him, and how the visit went.

In the group therapy that I was privileged to sit in on, Mrs France was focusing on getting the patients to make connections between actions and outcomes. She explained to me that the reason for the group is so that patients learn not to hold on to their own agony, to learn to listen to each other's problems, and to accept that others also have pain. She says that by listening to others' pain, they often learn to identify the origins of their own. Hearing another's story often prods one's memory, allowing forgotten matters to surface so they can be dealt with. The group helps them to learn to sympathize with each other. Since these patients have all committed violent crimes on other people, learning empathy is a prime priority. They learn it is admirable to have a soft side, as their prior life experiences had taught them only to be unsympathetic and tough.

Most importantly, Jenny France feels that by sharing their stories they develop language skills. Like Sue, they learn new vocabularies. Like Julia, they learn how to provide sufficient information so that co-conversational-ists can understand. They develop both listening and speech skills. The latter allow the patients to express themselves without resorting to violence. Just as Sue needs a new vocabulary to define herself, these men need vocabulary to articulate experience as well as to define themselves. Mrs France emphasized that they were not reasoned with as children. They were just belted, denigrated verbally and otherwise abused. The only response they had learned to make to frustrating experiences was violence.

Mrs France told me that most of the patients come into Broadmoor Hospital not able to express themselves at all verbally. The group often helps them out by saying 'Try to get it out' and 'We'll give you the words.' They learn that words are a better solution than violence.

The language-building skills Mrs France emphasizes include those of kindness, teaching patients to express sympathy and concern. She and the group, for instance, sympathize verbally with someone who is having bad dreams or poor reactions to medications. They verbally applaud the patient who has gone out of the hospital for a party and behaved socially appropriately. One patient was very proud that on a visit to his granddad, he was able to say 'No' politely to beer despite his granddad's insistence that he have some. He saw he could control his actions verbally, not argue, and not fight. Again, both Mrs France and the group applauded him, both verbally and kinesically. The latter included micromovements like head nodding in rhythm with the speaker's tale, a sure sign of what Erickson[5] calls *rhapsody* in conversation. Recall that this supportive, kind behaviour was observed in inmates at Broadmoor Hospital, a hospital for the crimi-nally insane. Each person in that group had committed a serious crime against at least one other person, but still had been able to learn kindness, and to achieve personal insights, by being skilfully taught to verbalize.

In sum, the speech therapist helped teach her patients, individually or in groups, new ways of looking at themselves, ways to deal with events verbally rather than physically, and how to interact politely. Politeness minimizes aggressive responses. Indeed, that is one reason all societies have politeness routines, to avoid confrontations. Jenny France literally taught her patients to speak their way to wellness, to a potentially more satisfying, socially fulfilling life. This was confirmed by the patients themselves.

In the group therapy session, at one point Mrs France asked how long a certain patient, less than 30 years old, had been in the hospital. He answered 'Eight years.' 'Eight years?' she replied. 'That's a good chunk of life.' He answered calmly, 'It's a different life,' whereupon a third party added seriously, 'It's like finishing school.' It was clear that this group understood the therapeutic process and appreciated its importance. To my knowledge, speech therapists in America do not do psychotherapy, but, as my experience with Jenny France and other speech therapists in the UK shows, their focus on language change fits in well with what we know of how people use language both to define themselves and to interact with the world. Moreover, other therapists can utilize the same techniques.

A therapeutic interview

The therapy sessions I observed at Broadmoor contrasted greatly with the one mentioned in Chapter 2 between a psychiatrist, Dr X.Y. and his client Helena. As was explained in the previous chapter, all information comes from Helena's diaries of the eight sessions she had with him. The fact that the therapist in this instance is a psychiatrist is not germane to what he did. That is, I wouldn't expect other psychiatrists to speak as he did. We have already examined from the vantage point of pragmatics how his use of sarcasm effected an accusation against the client. Any mental health professional could have done the same, just as any can treat their clients or patients with kindness and understanding.

Helena was a middle-aged, deeply depressed woman, secretly reduced to days in bed and non-stop crying which ceased only on the days she had to get up and get to work. While on her job, she was able to act competently, collapsing only when she returned home. Since her children were teenagers and her husband worked long hours, rarely were any of them home, enabling her to stay in her room undetected. Apparently, so far as her family and colleagues knew, she was a self-confident human being who had it all. She was educated, poised, maintained an enviable career, which she was at the top of, but balanced this by fulfilling her familial duties as a devoted mother of four, as well as a proper wife and a caring daughter. This, at least, is how she presented herself to the world, her family and herself. She always did the 'right' things. In light of theories of female depression, such as that described below, it must be emphasized that Helena strikes people as being articulate, outspoken and strong, albeit a traditional woman in carrying out her duties to her family.

Still, regardless of all her apparent successes, she had been deeply depressed for eight years before seeking psychiatric help. During that time, her family doctor prescribed anti-depressants for her. However, they had ceased to work. She presented herself to the psychiatrist as being depressed for no reason at all, and as having no problems. Dr X.Y.'s friendly and non-authoritarian manner made her decide to do therapy with him as her depression was becoming more and more debilitating especially now that pills alone couldn't help. On her second visit, she asked, 'Where should I begin?' to which he replied 'Wherever you want' To her own surprise, she found herself telling him about her childhood, a period of life which she had almost totally repressed. In Baars[6] and Chafe's[7] terms, her memories had simply not been activated since she abandoned her family at the age of 18 by eloping with a man they greatly disapproved of. Subsequently divorcing him, she eventually returned to her family and her interrupted college education.

Her childhood, it turned out, was a time of repeated violence against her person both by her father's battering and her mother's repeated harangues about what a terrible child she was. As she started to tell the story, more and more memories were activated. In the fourth therapy session Dr X.Y. shocked and offended Helena by his response to her offering (see pages 44–6).

By her choice of words in describing helping her brother, Helena's statement fits the speech event of a complaint.[8] The lexical selections leave no doubt: 'he made me type his papers'. The choice of made me indicates that her compliance was not wholly willing. She continues with 'Even if it was ...' The even underscores at the very least that she expected her therapist to agree with her that being awakened for this purpose was a strong imposition and evinced a disregard for her as a person. The fact that she 'had to get up,' further indicates coercion. Had to is a catenative verb auxiliary which has largely replaced must. Her selection of adjective to describe her brother's writing, botched up, certainly did not indicate admiration. She repeats that she 'had to literally decode', again indicating both coercion by the brother and that the chore was onerous. Her choice of the verb auxiliary must in 'what he must have meant' shows that her focus lay in her preserving his intended meaning, not in imposing her own so that he would get good grades. This is reinforced by her remarking that she was able to put it into 'understandable English'.

That she did this against her will and feeling put upon in the process is very evident both by her narrative sequence and her choice of words. Yet the therapist's comments made it seems as if he thought that she voluntarily did her brother's work even in the middle of the night, even though there could have been no conceivable payback for her to do this at all, much less under the imposed conditions. She did not present this as a good deed on her part, but as a clear burden.

Indeed, there was no need to mention these occurrences at all unless she was bragging or complaining. If it were the former, then why utilize words that reek of being compelled to act against her wishes and that stressed the difficulty of the task? Had she not been complaining, there would have been no need to speak of her disrupted sleep or to use verb forms which indicate coercion. Perhaps she indicated that she was able to decode the brother's convoluted prose because she was informing the therapist of her competence, but the complaint was still clear, and the situation clearly onerous. In the light of how Helena narrated these events, Dr X.Y.'s response is very puzzling indeed. Certainly he did not respond to her clear complaint, much less to the injustice of the demands placed upon her.

Moreover, as we shall see in Chapter 6, studies into how and when people tell stories show they do so to build their own egos, or to explore their present problems, not to present themselves as unworthy members of society. When asked, Helena said that it had never occurred to her, either then or later, that typing and editing her brother's papers could have been seen as cheating in any way, shape or manner. When the therapist responded as he did in, Helena described her reaction as feeling as if she had been punched in the stomach.

The client, perceived the therapist's response as a comment on her and her brother's lack of morality. Dr X.Y. was telling the client that she had cheated by aiding and abetting her brother in writing his papers for him. The therapist completely ignored the bizarre situation in which a young lady should be awakened in the middle of the night and feel as if it were her duty to shake the sleep out of her eyes, get dressed, and then decode page after page of her brother's obscure writing. Yet, this certainly raised important issues about Helena's position in her family. She was clearly inferior, at least in relation to her brother. Helena's account should also have raised questions about the dynamics of the family such as whether this position of inferiority was typical of her other familial relations. The psychiatrist also didn't question why the brother needed so much help in writing comprehensible essays. Had the therapist asked, he would have discovered that the brother went to a prestigious Ivy League college and did not require the sister's help in remaining near the top of his class except for the matter of writing papers, making his demands for his sister's help even more noteworthy. The alert therapist would have questioned why the brother needed such help and how the brother received the finished products. Had he done so, more information pertinent to the client's situation might have been forthcoming. For instance, the brother never thanked the Helena, nor gave any acknowledgment of her help. In fact, the brother was a diagnosed schizophrenic who couldn't write papers because of the opacity of his written language. Just as most speech-disordered schizophrenics start out speaking appropriately and then descend into various degrees of incoherence as they talk, the brother was able to write short paragraphs answering a question in a test. However, given the longer format of a term paper, his writing progressively dissolved into incoherence. Helena would figure out what his intentions were by the relatively coherent openings and had learned to interpret much of the rest. By asking him short questions as she edited his papers, she could garner what it was he was trying to communicate when the paper descended into gross incoherence.

There was one other question raised by Helena's story which might have cast light on her debilitating depression. Besides the questions which should have been asked about her family was another equally important one. Why had she become depressed so many years after these events? Rather than exploring the psychodynamics underlying this situation, the therapist completely cut off any more enquiry, including the relevance of Helena's past or present circumstances to her depression. Had he asked the correct questions, had he asked any questions at all, perhaps, the way would have been paved for discovering the underlying causes of Helena's depression. In fact, the therapist–client interview ended as fast as the patient could retreat from his office that day. About two weeks later, however, Helena, still in an almost unbearable depression, felt compelled to return to Dr X.Y., and said, at the outset of the interview:

> (2) Helena: About what I was telling you about my brother's papers. How is that any different from asking someone to read and comment on your paper before you hand it in?
> Dr X.Y. Ehhh
> (after this pause filler, he simply changed the topic completely)

Evidently, the therapist's original reaction had been preying on Helena's mind and she wanted to justify herself. We can see her again raising the topic of her brother's papers as an attempt to save her own face, to get the psychiatrist to view her in a better light; she wanted to vindicate herself to him. When he still didn't respond to this, Helena then truly felt he had a low estimation of her and her character and, certainly, that he had no interest in her or her problems. This reinforced her feelings of unworthiness, her feelings that, despite all that she had achieved, as a human being she was of no account. She ceased therapy with Dr X.Y. soon after this.

In fact, obviously, when Helena first mentioned the business of her brother's papers, besides complaining, she must have been raising a topic, and certainly not one that implicated her as a cheat. Therapy, after all, is not the confessional booth. As noted, she had started telling him about her childhood in the previous visits. She had already told the therapist of the physical and mental abuse she had suffered, abuse she had buried so deeply it had been forgotten. More precisely, it had not been consciously accessed for years. Narrating the childhood horrors reminded her of the incidents she had also buried for years about her duties to her brother.

The therapist, then, had a background in which to fit (1) and (2) above. Clearly, there had to be a connection between Helena's being maltreated as a child and the unreasonable demands made on her during her adolescence. One would think that the therapist's job at this point was at least to ask, 'Why?' 'Why would your brother feel he could wake you up?' 'Why did you do his papers for him?' 'What did your parents think of your getting up in the middle of the night to do his work for him?' The answer to the last alone would have yielded important information. Helena claims that the parents would have been angry had she not helped the brother, although he was never expected to help her in any way. Helena's story in (1) leant itself to many questions, all important to the therapeutic situation, all important to uncovering the causes of her depression.

In terms of immediate outcomes, the result of her encounter was that Helena left therapy and continued trying to go it alone for several months, all the while suffering from deep depression and emotional pain. Perhaps because of her background, Helena didn't blame the therapist. She simply assumed she deserved his scorn. In fact, moralistic sarcasm had been a big weapon among the members of her family, and a major way of putting everybody down, in and out of the family. The psychiatrist appeared to do to her what her family had always done.

Two years later, when she dared undergo therapy again, so devastated had she been by this first experience, she tentatively recounted the story in (1) above to a different therapist, Dr L.G. His responses were quite different. In fact, he asked many of the questions I mentioned above, especially those involving her place in the family.

First, Dr. L.G. indignantly exclaimed

Why did you think you had to wake up to do something like that? Even once, much less all during his college career?

This, of course, opened up the entire field of this family's dysfunctional operations. Because he asked the right questions, questions which in no way seemed to blame Helena or impugn her character, she was truly led to re-author her life through therapy. For instance, by the therapist's creating a warm interactive environment, Helena was able to remember more about her father's constantly beating her throughout her childhood and adolescence. These beatings shamed her, made her feel she was highly unworthy and deserved such treatment, a not uncommon assumption by abused people. Except for three sessions with Dr X.Y., she had never told anyone about this abuse and herself never thought of it consciously. By allowing Helena to remember, to re-feel, and, belatedly, to grieve, Dr L.G. was also able to establish with her that the beatings were her father's shame, not hers. It was he who had erred. There was nothing she had done to deserve such treatment. Once she realized this, she had success-fully rewritten part of her life story.

Therapy itself is an interactional achievement. It achieves what it does by skilful questioning, non-judgmental listening, encouraging the client to keep narrating his or her life, and, of course, interpreting what is recounted, linking and relinking it to different facets of experience. We shall address the mechanisms by which this is achieved after we have examined depression itself.

Through his skilled questioning, his careful and caring listening, and acute interpretations and by helping her to make connections between events and feelings, Dr L.G. and Helena were able to root out other causes of her depression. The importance of interconnecting narratives in the work of psychotherapy should not be ignored,[9] for it is the connection, usually performed by the therapist, sometimes by the client, which explicates the meaning of events. It also shows recurrent themes in ostensibly different narratives, themes which, in themselves, may be highly revealing.

By listening to and encouraging her narratives, Dr L.G. created an atmosphere in which Helena could finally activate the memories of her early years, memories which impinged directly on the current status of her life in that they influenced her later interpersonal relations. These were characterized by Helena's feeling that she had to satisfy every whim of her family, but never ask anything of them. Because of this, later in life, she was paralysed in the face of disciplining her brood and in even thinking of asking her husband to partake in child-raising or running the home. Recall that she, all this while, sustained a full-time demanding job. Helena was also finally able to unload the feelings of anger and resentment that were lurking below the shame, and to admit her virtual loathing of her parents. Nothing surprised her so much as having such feelings, never before consciously thought, much less said.

With Dr L.G.'s help, Helena was also able to remember the non-stop verbal abuse of her mother. Virtually daily, her mother indulged in harangues about what an unworthy creature Helena was. The mother claimed that she herself was virtually a superhuman paragon who had, from her early teens, run her own mother's household. Furthermore, Helena's mother emphasized, she didn't 'sit around and play bridge all day the way other women did'. Rather, she worked at a hard and demeaning job as a shoe salesperson in a local department store. Undoubtedly these harangues reinforced the mother's bruised ego, but probably not as much as they bruised Helena's. From an early age, Helena was supposed to keep house, do the ironing and laundry and even cook meals. If she did these chores well, there was no comment, but if there was any lapse, it provoked an elongated rebuke from her mother.

Never once could Helena evoke a childhood memory of being praised or of being touched other than in anger. Added to this, although she was the younger child by eleven months, Helena was expected to care for her brother, give him meals and run his errands. In early adolescence, he had a severe psychotic break. Rather than consign him to the local mental institution, the parents elected to keep him at home with Helena as his caregiver. This was why she had to edit his papers for him. Even when in a non-psychotic state, the brother's writings suffered from schizophrenic speech disorder. His sentences were so torturous, his wording so obscure, and filled with extraneous matter combined with persistent repetitions, that he needed an editor.

Fortunately, Helena was always a good student. The good grades she achieved at school were partially by her own talents, as her therapist pointed out but, as she herself recalled, partially to avoid the beatings that poor grades would have yielded. In any event, school successes were also the one positive ego experience in her young life, eventually enabling her to complete college and even graduate school.

One question remained, however. Why did this debilitating depression express itself now when she was at the pinnacle of her career? She was long free of her parents. Better yet, the arduous duties of getting a doctorate while she was mothering young children were behind her. Either of these demand a great deal of mental and physical strength. Engaging in both at the same time as Helena did spoke of extraordinary self-control and energy. If her earlier years alone were what eventually led her to crack, one would think it would have been in graduate school, a time when judgmental criticism is especially concentrated, and one which coincided with the hectic young-mothering years. At the time of this telling, the children were all adolescents.

After Helena's early divorce, she married an affable man, one very unlike her father, and produced four children whom she raised with loads of physical affection and a minimum of discipline. As affable as her husband was, however, he left the entire raising of the children and running of the household to Helena, even when she held down a job equal to his in workload and money earned. When the children abused her verbally in his presence, he did not correct them. She did not even think of overtly questioning this as she had been raised to do it all by herself anyhow. At least her husband neither beat nor harangued her, nor did he demand subservience in any way. In fact, he never criticized her in any way. Blessedly, he didn't even expect her to wait on him. If anything, he waited on her, at least to the extent of bringing her morning coffee in bed. Compared to her birth family, her married one was vastly superior, although exhausting.

Despite the notorious obnoxiousness of adolescents in our society, Dr. L.G. never asked about the children. Had he, Helena might have verbalized what she could barely bring herself to think about: her children's behaviour. Now the only major assaults on her ego were those made by her adolescent children who were rude, demanding, sloppy, lazy, and extremely critical of her. It is easy to think that her early experiences had made her excessively sensitive to their slightest adolescent slurs, so that she was perceiving only the worst. However, upon questioning, she admitted to me that they even called her 'bitch' and 'cunt' when she tried to control them. To her, their behaviour was not only unbearably rude, but inexplicable. She had been, in her eyes, a permissive, affectionate, and loving mother, and had an idealized vision of how her children should speak and behave to her. Idealized, that is, in so far as she never expected to be referred to with such vulgarity, rudeness and lack of overt affection. She expected that, since she had raised them so differently from the way her parents raised her, they would just love her and be affectionate to her, like families in the movies of her childhood. It is entirely possible that the reason she had such a bevy to begin with is that she was trying to capture a loving, family situation, one denied her in childhood, but, she thought, attainable with her own children.

Some therapists might feel that something in Helena herself evoked such deprecatory treatment. That is, the victim caused her own victimization, but this is too pat, too easy and lets everyone, including the therapists, off the hook. They need seek no further for answers. Actually, to explain her children's behaviour, one must first look to society itself and prevalent attitudes and language. The language adolescents have been using for the past two decades or so is loaded with formerly taboo words. *Fuck* and *fucking* are favourite lexical items, and *bitch*, *ho*, *slut* and even *cunt* as designations for females are not unusual. Songs aimed at adolescents are rife with such language combined with defiant, rebellious attitudes towards older generations. Surely these linguistic facts about adolescence supply some explanation for the children's nastiness. This was the cultural climate for her children. Consequently, they probably didn't perceive that their language was as serious or demeaning as their mother felt it to be. Clearly, some family counselling was in order for Helena and her children, but this possibility was not even raised in her therapy.

The major point to this discussion is that the therapist must always be ready to understand behaviours in sociocultural terms as well as in individual historical terms. Whatever Helena and her husband did wrong, it was exacerbated by the social climate surrounding adolescents in Western societies.

As with her father's beatings and her mother's carping, Helena's response to the children was deep shame, a feeling of basic unworthiness. This, her children's behaviour, Helena was too ashamed to share spontaneously with Dr L.G. It may even be that she could not separate the feelings of shame from her feelings of depression. The degree to which shame underlies depression is rarely mentioned, even by those who study it, like Gilligan[10] and Jack. The degree to which mothers feel shame by their children's misbehaviour is also too often unspoken.

In any event, the therapist, L.G., didn't think to enquire about her role as mother or her children's behaviour at such a notoriously difficult time in their lives. At best, mothering is taken very much for granted in our society and, at worst, it is a devalued activity; hence, phrases like 'just a housewife' or 'stay-at-home mother'. Socially we see how disvalued parenting is when we see the scandal of our foster care system. We pay a pittance for such services when, in reality, foster parents should be well-trained professionals who receive appropriate compensation for their work. This is a symptom of how society sees child-raising. Since mothers are considered the prime child rearers, the devaluing of this role spreads to them or, perhaps, it is devalued because it is seen as women's work. Consequently, what the therapist did not see, indeed was barely conscious of, was how Helena's current home life, specifically her children's active behaviour and her husband's passive shunting of responsibility, psychologically repeated her early experiences. The therapist did not help Helena to see that her husband, as amiable as he was, was unfair in his failure to assume responsibility for the children. That issue never really came up in three years of therapy. Given the sensitivity and astuteness of the therapist in other instances, this is a curious failing, until one considers society's traditional expectations of parenthood. It is only relatively recently that fathers have been considered liable for their children's upbringing beyond providing ample income for it. Therapists, too, are products of society and its values; thus they can be blind to its underlying assumptions even when these are damaging to a client.

Still, with Dr L.G., Helena did learn how damaging her birth family had been to her ego, and that their downgrading her as a person was one underlying cause of her depression. She learned that she was a valuable human being who had accomplished a prodigious amount. The therapist helped her by showing her the injustice visited upon her in her early years. That she was reliving disparagement, now by her children, was never mentioned in therapy, nor did Helena make the connection at that time, although, later, on her own, with the help of a woman's diary-reading group, she was able to. This disparagement also may have had a heightened effect because in her career as a scholar, her work was always being critiqued and criticized.[11]

More broadly, she also couldn't see that she should have insisted upon her husband's taking equal responsibility for housework and child care because she felt that she was living up to society's expectations of her. We shall see this phenomenon again when we meet Meg in Chapter 6. Raising children and keeping a house is a mother's job even if she has another job, especially if opting for a career is perceived as her own choice. Helena had a husband. He did have a career. If she, too, had a career, then it was her choice and had to be added to her wifely duties, a psychically and physically exhausting combination. Note that, in this view, the money she contributed to the family by her outside work did not assume the same value as the husband's who was, after all, supposed to be the breadwinner. Her earnings were treated as incidental to her decision not to assume the traditional stay-at-home role. The irony in this case was that Helena made at least as much money as her husband did, and often more.

In sum, the therapist, Helena, and even her husband were all blinded by background and society. Her response was depression, especially because of the problems she had with her children, problems even her therapists failed to perceive or ask about. Helena herself did not perceive how her children exacerbated her depression until after many years of therapy and introspection. As we shall see below, this last, the role of children in a woman's depression, seems to be ignored in the main, even by researchers into female depression, like Dana Jack.

Depression

Jack[12] claims that 'The rate of depression is twice as high for women as for men in the United States and in most Western societies'. She attributes this to the fact that women suffer from *Silencing the Self*, the title of her book. I must point out that this doesn't mean that depression actually afflicts women more than men. The actual number of men who suffer from depression is unknown because men do not seek therapeutic help as readily as women do. Depression may be expressed differently by each gender. Women are given more leave by society to 'take to their beds' and to cry. Helena, for instance, reported crying for hours on end, the tears just pouring down. Men can't do this. Surely, however, it is significant that men are far more successful at suicide than women. Women try and fail. Men succeed. Perhaps that is the because of the degree to which men have no outlet to express depression in Western society.

In any event, Jack[13] feels that a woman is more susceptible to depression because 'inequality mutes her ability to communicate directly about her needs'. This is because Western society devalues dependence on others and women are seen as being dependent, requiring personal attachments. They are not autonomous. Our social ideal,[14] derived from capitalism and American mythology, is the lone cowboy, the hero, and 'the man who makes it on his own'. This is harmful for men and completely invalidates traditional female roles. According to this view, one shouldn't need relationships, but by her very nature the female of the species if she elects to be a wife and mother must depend upon relationships. So must children. Jack notes that Freud's own description of depression, the identification of the ego with an abandoned object, assumes that a healthy adult lives independently of and unaltered by relations, and that depression is caused by inability to detach from a relationship. Freud didn't see depression as arising from an inability to connect. It seems to me that the masculine ideal of the lone hero, autonomous, needing nobody but himself actually describes an asocial, pathological individual.[15] Such an ideal is as damaging to the men it purports to serve as to women, who are virtually excluded from it by their social roles.

Jack[16] does mention that 'research findings regarding the importance of relationships to mental health, as well as theory regarding the central role of attachments throughout life' shows that it is unfair to deprecate women as dependent. What Jack does not acknowledge is that men are silenced as equally as women. Men cannot admit their dependence on relationships, although these are as important to them as they are to women. Yet, traditional Freudian psychiatry has consistently characterized depression as 'pathologic dependency' and as 'submissive, manipulative, ... piteous...[attempts to maintain relationships]'[17] On such a view, Helena's feelings for her children and, earlier, for her parents might be seen as a form of dependence but, in truth, her birth family depended on her, and children, by their very nature, must depend upon their parents. Co-dependency reinforced by affection is the natural human family condition. Its absence is abnormal and a legitimate cause of depression.

Linde[18] and others who have studied how people create narratives of their lives have demonstrated that one underlying factor is always for a person to present him or herself as a worthwhile member of society who fulfils society's expectations. Proof of this, clearly, is that one is loved and accepted by others, in and out of the family. One who is rejected, or feels as if he or she is, suffers greatly in self-esteem. Jack[19] quotes Gilligan as saying 'goodness is understood as conformity to social norms and values, as fulfilling the obligations and functions of the roles one occupies: wife/mother/daughter/woman'. Note that the first three of these involve caring, self-sacrificing and hard work for others. Of all of these, being a good mother demands the most. Furthermore, it is expected that a woman will bring up her children 'right', and if they turn out poorly, becoming drug addicts or school dropouts, then it is her fault. Even if the children do achieve, if they are rude or nasty to their mothers, or never willingly visit them, then many expect that the mother deserves it. Complaining about one's mother and every mistake she ever made is virtually a cottage industry in the Western world.

Yet Jack almost completely ignores motherhood as a cause of depression except when discussing how daughters learn to be submissive from mothers who were 'doormats'[20] or were otherwise poor role models. Like Freud, with whom she specifically disagrees in many ways, and like American society as well, Jack sees dysfunction in women as the fault of their mothers. Jack's main concern with motherhood is the way that daughters learn to identify with their mothers, and how this identification causes the daughters' depression.[21] It does not seem to have occurred to her that the mothers she was talking about were themselves depressed or trying as hard as they could to be good women as society dictates that role. Never does she look at mothering from the vantage of being a mother.

Indeed, Jack developed a metric for determining the degree of a woman's depression which doesn't mention motherhood or parenthood at all. She calls this test the Silencing the Self Scale.[22] Respondents circle a number from 1 to 5 according to the degree to which he or she agrees with the given statements, 31 in all. Sample questions from this scale are (numbering hers):

1. I don't speak my feelings in an intimate relationship because no one else will look out for me.

3.   Caring means putting the other person's needs before my own.
18. When my partner's needs or opinions conflict with mine, rather than
     asserting my own point of view I usually end up agreeing with
     him/her.

In this scale, eight questions specifically referred to a partner, and nine
others referred specifically to 'a relationship', meaning one between two
adults. Four others were starred, as not typical of the female role, such as

*8. When my partner's needs and feelings conflict with my own, I always
     state mine clearly.
*11. In order to feel good about myself, I need to feel independent and
     self-sufficient.

The others, like (3) above, did refer to a female's role as caregiver, but
none directly mentioned children and the mother–child relationship. Yet,
as most mothers will verify, the depth and strength of the mother–child
bond, at least from the mother's view, is unparalleled and quite different
from that even for a passionately loved partner. Moreover, failing as a
mother is far more socially condemned than is a failure as a partner. A
mother can't leave her children without social reprobation, but she can
leave her partner.

The one time Jack[23] considers mothers apart from their function as bad
role models, she quotes someone else as noting that children 'become the
misdirected targets of her [a wife's] unexpressed rage towards her
spouse'. No supporting proof is given for this generalization and nowhere
does Jack mention or quote anybody as showing how children may
become misdirected targets of their father's unexpressed rage towards
others, although the statistics on child abuse to the point of killing young
children point to fathers as frequent culprits in mistreatment of their
young. Jack, under the guise of feminism, reinforces traditional anti-
female gender attitudes.

There is no way to understand a mother's depression without also
understanding her relationships with her children and also understanding
that if that relationship is difficult, it may not wholly be her fault, although
society and mythology both reinforce that it is. Jackie Kennedy Onassis
was often quoted as saying that if a woman bungles raising her children,
she is a failure in life. Freud, of course, made the mother the prime villain
in any problems her children had later in life. Bateson,[24] in a theory which
still has adherents, although it has no supporting data at all, blames
mothers for schizophrenia. He claims mothers who don't love their
children put them in a double-bind situation such that if the child says
truthfully, 'You don't love me', the mother both denies it and punishes the
child; hence, the child never learns to communicate, causing schizophrenia. It is amazing how farfetched researchers have been willing to go

to blame mothers when there were and are no scientific bases for the conclusions they wanted to find.

In a case like Helena's, her depression was aggravated because there wasn't any person she could admit to that she was having problems with her children. She couldn't complain about them, either, for to complain would be, in effect, an admission of how terrible they were. If therapy, in collusion with social norms, blames mothers, then how can mothers blame their children? No matter how successful she was in her job, Helena felt that she was a failure by society's standards. This, of course, made her feel ashamed.

Apart from her shame, as deep a shame as being a battered child was, part of her necessary image as a competent career woman depended upon her being seen as a good, competent mother, and good mothers don't have nasty children. Even a strong, articulate, intelligent, career woman is silenced when it comes to her role as mother. None of this should be read as meaning that fathers are unaffected by their children. Fathers aren't immune either. They, too, can feel depressed over their children, and they are as silenced as women are. It is ironic that scholars focus on the silencing of a woman's voice, without perceiving the silencing of men, especially in their personal lives.

During one session, Dr X.Y. asked Helena what it was like to be a teacher, but he didn't ask her what it was like being a mother, although the latter was certainly as forceful a factor in her life as her teaching was. The more sensitive therapist, Dr L.G., never brought up or seriously considered her relationship with her children. When she tentatively broached the subject to L.G., he dismissed the subject by saying 'To have raised four children who are finishing school, can hold down jobs and form long-lasting loving relations is an achievement in these days'. Then he changed the subject. Helena's point was not going to be about her children's successes, but on how they interacted with her, and how painful she found their behaviour towards her.

It seems to me that every therapist should delve deeply into the mother–child relations of depressed females who are mothers, and the father–child relationship of men. Parenthood is as important a facet of someone's emotional states as their relation with their partner is. Certainly, Helena's depression had many causes, but its onset and severity coincided with adolescence – her children's.

One of the anonymous readers of an earlier manuscript of this book questioned whether or not uncovering the cause of depression helps. With good therapy, it can help in at least three ways. First, and most simply, it makes anybody feel better to share their pain, to let off steam, to tell a non-judgmental sympathetic person their woes. That is just human. Second, a skilful therapist can assure the depressed person that he or she is not having unique problems. They are not unworthy because they have such problems; others are in the same boat. That is often a relief. Finally, they can devise steps for alleviating the conditions which cause the depression. This brings us to the next section.

Behavioural-cognitive therapy

Jack[25] rightly deplores the psychoanalytic dictum that, because of the defensive manoeuvres of the unconscious ego, people's own explanations for their emotions can't be trusted. Thus, in Freudian-based analyses an expert, an outsider, becomes the trusted interpreter of the self. Jack says all such views negate the patients' own experiences and teach distrust for what they have to say.

I heartily agree with Jack, but listening to the patient involves non-judgmental, non-theoretically biased interviewing. Moreover, the therapist must be prepared to ask questions about all facets of a client's life. It is not enough to ask, 'What was your mother like?' One must also ask 'What is it like being a mother?' 'How difficult do you find your children?' One must ask of a man as well as a woman 'How alone do you feel?' 'Do you depend on anyone?' Preconceived theorizing is no better in a therapy which allows the client to speak of his or her own experiences than it is in Freudian or other belief systems.

Helena's illness seems to be a good candidate for a revised version of the talking cure: behavioural-cognitive therapy. This is a 'talk' therapy aimed at changing self-defeating patterns of thought and behaviour. It has been championed as requiring far fewer visits, as few as 12–16, than more traditional therapies.[26] It considers itself different from other therapies because it does not rely upon digging up childhood memories. Rather, it focuses on present problems. However, behavioural-cognitive therapy, too, can suffer from preconceived narrowness. For instance, consider Jack's description of depression and its treatment:

> People who are depressed may live by the unspoken assumption that nobody loves them, or that everything they try fails ... They will see their entire lives through this dark prism, overemphasizing the events that support their negative views and filtering out those that contradict them. The therapist helps them identify those thoughts and replace them with a more accurate picture.

Depressive individuals are seen as exaggerating the negative aspects of experience. One practitioner of behavioural-cognitive therapy quoted by Freyer said it is a misconception that cognitive therapy says you shouldn't feel bad when bad things happened, but you should just feel bad, not depressed. This cognitive therapist says that you shouldn't feel depressed because depression implies helplessness. Here is a conundrum. Since depression by definition makes you feel bad, and feeling bad makes you depressed, how does one distinguish between the two? Even if you just feel bad, your ability to function is diminished. Furthermore, telling a depressed person to look at the bright side of things is tantamount to telling him or her to 'Buck up! Things aren't so bad!' But what if the picture they have is, in the main, accurate? Many depressed people are depressed because their lives are depressing. Besides, even if there are good things in their lives, they still have to deal with what is depressing them.

Rather than assuming that there must be overlooked bright spots that could somehow offset the depressing situations, the behavioural-cognitive therapist should be asking questions like: 'What is upsetting you?' 'Why is this happening?' 'Who are the important people in your life, and how are they behaving towards you? 'How angry are you at the person(s) who cause you to feel this way?' 'What have you tried to do to alter the other's action or inaction?' 'How stressful is your job?' 'How much criticism or negative feedback do you get from co-workers or bosses?' Such questions can fit in with behavioural-cognitive therapy or any other kind of therapy. Even in behavioural-cognitive therapy the onus is on the interviewer to get at the problem and to do so with no preconceptions such as 'things really aren't as bad as they seem'. They may not be, or they may be. That is what it is up to the therapy to discover.

When questioned, Helena did admit that her children were not unremittingly rude and obnoxious to her. Their attacks were, to her, unpredictable, and when they did occur, were terrible. If a therapist, behavioural-cognitive or other, had asked about her children, while acknowledging her pain, the therapist could have tried to get her at least not to dwell solely on their adolescent outbursts, as she was clearly doing.

Her treatment should have included techniques to alleviate outbursts, something as simple as refusing to give them an audience by merely walking out of a room when she was treated rudely. A behavioural plan should have been set up which denied her children privileges when they misbehaved, combined with making them earn points by good behaviour for the things they wanted. This is hardly a new technique, and wasn't so when Helena was in therapy, but since nobody bothered to find out that she was suffering from her children, nobody advised her what to do about it. The irony of this situation is that in her community, unbeknown to her, there was a family service in which a team of behavioural and clinical therapists visited the home and worked directly with the families *in situ*. Since Helena's health insurance paid for this, it would have cost nothing.

The therapist could have discussed the fact that adolescents today do act this way, and that her 1950s Hollywood version of families is not reality. This wouldn't have taken away the hurt each attack caused her, nor would it have shown her how her childhood experiences heightened her sensitivity to personal affronts, but it might possibly have helped somewhat to get her to concentrate on the few positive experiences she could have with her children at this time, as well as to realize that they would grow up and, presumably, their repugnant behaviour would then subside. Many an obnoxious teenager turns out to be a loving daughter or son when he or she grows up. One hopes Helena's will do, too. If she fears hers won't, then she could be led to the realization that, at least, she wouldn't have to have them at home, and she could try to build a life in which her dealings with them did not play such an important role in her life. Even if they weren't giving her trouble, she should be preparing for such a time as children do leave home and do have their own adult lives to live.

Any therapy, no matter its label, might have taught her to think of times when her children were not nasty to her. She could have been encouraged to think of some good interactions with them, if any occurred. Since humour defuses most situations, she could be encouraged to joke with her children or make light of their outbursts. Instead of dissolving in tears when insulted, she could make humorous remarks like, 'It must be awful to be a prince and have to live in this hovel' or 'How awful it is for a princess to be raised by clods like us.' or she could acknowledge the teenager's angst, saying 'I'm sorry something so bad happened to you today that you're acting this way. But is it fair to take it out on me?' Then, calmly, she should go on about her business. It would also have accomplished a great deal if she had learned to walk away from verbal abuse without responding to it, thus making argumentation impossible.

However, as this example shows, the therapist of any school, behavioural-cognitive or not, has to beware of one thing. Before urging a client to think that they are overlooking the bright spots, the therapist had better be sure there are some good times with the bad. Otherwise, the situation would seem even worse to the client.

There are no pat platitudes in family or personal therapy, although, as we shall shortly see, platitudes play a big role in groups which seek to change behaviour such as alcoholism or drugtaking. These groups are concerned only with the here and now, and the focus is on the participant himself or herself with one overriding goal: getting him or her to stop drinking or using drugs. Multi-faceted relations with family or partners aren't the focus. In essence, anti-addiction therapies are geared to change one aspect of behaviour, addiction, which in itself causes problems with all other relationships. Thus it is inevitable that speech forms are used differently and for different purposes than in therapy aimed at individuals with problems that are not caused by self-abuse of drugs or alcohol.

Therapy as speech event

It is clear from the above that therapy itself is a **speech event**, a situation calling forth particular ways of speaking. It is an unusual speech event, however, in that it overlaps considerably with the stuff of ordinary conversation: informing, commenting, anecdote telling, questioning and answering about one's personal life. Like good conversation, a good therapy session achieves what Erickson[27] terms **rhapsody**, a stitching together of a conversation between speaker and hearer. Erickson was not talking about the therapeutic situation, but his observations are apropos.

In ordinary conversation, when speakers are all 'in synch' with each other, Erickson and Schulz[28] claim, the conversation can be set to a metronome. Movements, whether micromovements like head nodding, or larger ones like legcrossing, are synchronized with utterances[29] and eye contact, the rhythmic looking at and then looking away between conversants is similarly subconsciously orchestrated. Topics just seem to 'come up' and there is no concern about relevancy to a higher purpose. Information may be imparted, but the conversation is not limited to the getting and giving of such information, much less to interpreting it. In addition, such conversing is based upon equality of interactants, and therapy is not.

Although therapy may achieve rhapsody at times – and remember, not all casual conversation achieves it either – all therapy is different from conversation in several important respects, not the least of which is the inequality of the participants. Also, in conversation the same restraints on topic raising usually apply to all participants. It is outré, for instance, in American society to ask another adult how much money he or she makes or has, or how much he or she weighs. Certainly, one can't usually ask a co-conversationalist if he or she masturbates or performs oral sex no matter how much rhapsody is achieved.

In contrast, in therapy, the client is far more constrained from raising topics with the therapist than the therapist is with the client. Clients, in general, cannot ask the therapist anything about his or her personal life or daily activities, past or present. The therapist, obviously, can and must ask about such matters and, if the client raises a topic, then the therapist has the right to ask even deeper questions about it. The therapist has far more rights and far fewer constraints in questioning in all aspects of the thera-peutic situation than does the client.

Then, too, whereas ordinary conversation has no necessary time or event limitations, the therapeutic situation is severely constrained by time. The client has an appointment consisting of so many minutes. All inter-acting is done within the time set aside for him or her. It is assumed that all anecdotes or questioning by either party are relevant to the problems of the client. Still, as Ferrara[30] shows, therapy is social interaction, and good therapy may achieve a synchronicity of its own, evincing rapport between therapist and client.

Ferrara[31] sees therapy as belonging to the speech event of **consultation** when one person goes to a specialist to receive assistance in planning future behaviour or action. Although this definition certainly encompasses going to a lawyer or financial adviser or even a physician, it does not quite include therapy in all its aspects. Often the therapist specifically eschews advising on future courses of action. The client consults the therapist in order to alleviate present symptoms, such as anxiety or depression, and to uncover past experiences which have led to present problems. Still, in the main, Ferrara I believe is correct. In many respects, therapy is *sui generis*, but in other ways it belongs to a set of consultations. It is probably most accurate to recognize that each type of consultation: legal, financial or medical, follows its own rules.

Joint production

Psychotherapy is a joint production between therapist and client. Ferrara[32] specifically shows that nothing illustrates this more than the amount and kinds of repetition and completions that inhere in the process, and that both repetition and completions are a vital part of achieving and maintaining rapport in therapy. She claims that 'repetitions of the words of others ... shows that people often construct their discourse out of bits and pieces of others' talk, ... **jointly building discourse**' (emphasis mine). It seems to me that the repetitions in and of themselves form cohesiveness between speakers' contributions to the interactions, as well as further rapport between them, by acting as a way of saying 'I understand you. I sympathize with you. I'm on your wavelength.' By repeating another's words, one is validating them as worth building upon.

Ferrara divides repetitions into two forms: **echoing** and **mirroring**. Of these, the first is especially important in therapy. Echoing constitutes a repetition often by the client, with appropriate changes in pronominals, matching a downward intonation used in the original statement. Ferrara[33] gives the example:

> Marian (therapist):   You're scared of men ↘
> Sharon (client):   I'm scared of men ↘
>
> [arrows indicate direction of voice, here falling]

Note that if Sharon had used an upward intonation, the meaning would have been something like 'You must be kidding. I'm not scared of men.' Had the therapist used an upward intonation, then she would have been asking, 'Are you scared of men?' However, the therapist's statement presents this as a fact she has figured out about Sharon, and Sharon's matching of words and downward intonation functions as an emphatic agreement. Notice that Sharon could have just said, 'Yes, I am,' but this doesn't begin to have the force of her agreement by echoing. Ferrara points out also that echoing not only shows emphatic agreement, but also demonstrates empathy,[34] the ability to take the other's point of view.

Although Ferrara claims that echoing is usually client-generated, that is, the client does the echoing to indicate agreement and empathy, it can as easily be therapist-generated. Had Sharon been the first to say 'I'm scared of men,' and the therapist had echoed with 'You're scared of men' with the same downward contour, then the therapist would have shown exceptional empathy with the client, as well as affirmation of her insight. Besides establishing rhapsody between the therapist and client, such therapist-generated echoing can encourage the client to continue to analyse on his or her own. The client can naturally feel that the therapist is on his or her side.

Ferrara[35] also demonstrates that another kind of iteration with a downward contour, what she calls *mirroring*, serves another important purpose in the therapeutic interview. Mirroring doesn't repeat the entire statement as echoing does. Nor is it contiguous with the original statement as echoing is. Rather, a word or phrase is plucked from a recently previous statement and serves, she shows, as *an indirect request*[36] for the client to continue. Ferrara postulates that such mirroring is designed to increase the clients' awareness by teaching them to listen to their own words and consider their meaning as they expand on the semantic content.

One of Ferrara's examples again cites the therapist Marian and the client Sharon. Sharon says she no longer feels 'in danger of exploding' at her job and that she is hardly in the office any more. The therapist goes back to to the phrase 'in danger of exploding', repeating it in a thoughtful, even tone. This is a way of saying, 'Hold on! What did you mean by you used to feel in danger of exploding?'

Echoing is more emphatic than a non-iterated response, but mirroring is a less emphatic way of saying 'Tell me more.' Again, it seems to me, that repeating the client's words, even though the result is less overt, increases cohesiveness and bonding between therapist and client. Ferrara claims that mirroring is usually therapist-generated. That is, the therapist mirrors the client's remarks as a way of encouraging the latter to explicate further.

Repetition

Repetition occurs in therapy in other ways. Chief among these are the retellings of the same story or of different stories with the same themes. Space here does not permit even an adequate summary of Ferrara's[37] analyses of 'Retellings in Therapeutic Discourse' except for one important factor. The therapist can encourage such retellings by using the usual sounds and words to encourage a speaker, such as 'Mmmm', 'Uhuh', 'Really?' and the like. It has long been known in sociolinguistics that because such backchannelled cues not only show interest, even sympathy, they increase the length and depth of the speaker's response. Such cueing is often accompanied by head bobbing in synch with the speaker's rhythms and inclining the body towards the speaker, both of which also serve as signalling involvement in what the speaker has to say. One factor in cross-gender communication, for instance, is that women encourage men to speak by such cueing, but men don't encourage women. Thus men, inadvertently or not, by not uttering sounds of interest, dampen women's tellings. Perhaps the male therapist has to be especially aware of the dampening effect of just sitting silently. In therapy, it is especially important to encourage retellings because often they are what illustrate and give insight into problems. Subsequent retellings expand upon and give more insights. They allow the therapist – or the client – eventually to see certain theme(s). The very fact that stories get retold shows their importance to the therapeutic situation.

Not surprisingly, perhaps, Dr X.Y., discussed above, Helena's first therapist, did not realize this. Helena reports that she complained to him several times that her husband paid no attention to her or the children, recounting several stories over the course of three or four interviews to illustrate this point. Finally, Dr X.Y., rather than tying together the themes of these narratives, said, 'You keep complaining about your husband. Yet you stay with him.' Actually, her retellings had at least three possible meanings. One, a question of whether her life would be better if she left her husband, certainly a topic to be discussed with care. Second, if she should leave him, why was she so loathe to? What did it say about her that she remained with someone who was so indifferent to her and her pain? Or, third, what could she do to make her husband more aware? The therapist's response did not invite exploration of any of these issues. Again, we see that therapy is a joint production. What gets elaborated on, what problems get an airing, and what revelations come forth is a matter of therapist encouragement of the client's contribution.

Another important facet of the joint production inherent in therapy is that of one speaker completing the sentence of another. Not surprisingly, this happens in ordinary conversation as well. It can be a factor in rhapsody between two speakers, showing one is so in tune with the other's words that one can guess what the other is going to say next. For instance,

> Ben: ... They must've had some type of a <u>showing</u>.– A camper show or uhm – flea market,
> Ethel: at the great big drive in theater
> Ben: or they mighta had a swap meet ...

Sacks[38] gives this as an example of the intimacy of 'spouse talk'. Note that the entire co-ordinate sentence is truly a joint production, with Ethel's 'at the great big drive in theater' a prepositional phrase acting as an adverbial of place to Ben's first utterance, and Ben's co-ordinating 'or they mighta had a swap meet' picking up without missing a beat. Notice that the structures each produces occur at natural syntactic breaks, and each produces phrases and clauses that complement what the other said. This is a true joint production and shows the intimacy of the two. Although, as with all language functions, completions may serve more than one purpose,[39] here we consider them only in their function of rhapsody, 'fine tuning of thoughts and words between discourse participants'.[40] They are possible only if the second speaker is paying very close attention to the first one's every word since the completion must be in the appropriate grammatical form. Ferrara[41] found such completions both by therapists and clients. She says[42] that such completions may show genuine empathy engendered by the therapist–client relationship, but that they may also be used as a 'means of creating empathy or the appearance of it'. She gives as examples the client's statement that her boss is beginning to deal with her now. The therapist picks up on the 'now' and completes the client's statement with 'now he thinks he might lose you'. The therapist actually starts to say 'now...' just as the client says it. Another example is from a therapist, Gerald's, commenting that Wilma, the client, talks about someone in a certain way. As he is talking, saying that she talks about someone in... Wilma breaks in and finishes the prepositional phrase started by Gerald by saying '...a negative way'.

Ferrara[43] does warn that completing another's utterance as a social practice can be a dangerous (her word) practice because 13 per cent of the time, four out of 30 instances in her corpus, either clients or therapists, rejected the other's completions. The fact that we don't read each other's minds perfectly in all situations is not shocking news, especially in complex interactions like therapy sessions. Still, this does not negate the bonding inherent in even attempting to complete what the other says. It still shows that the therapist is listening closely and is trying to remain in tune. Of course, like all good things, completing another's sentences, if done too often, can be read as impatience on the part of the therapist, or that the client is not being given a chance to express him or herself.

In sum

This chapter has shown that the rules of ordinary social interaction often must be obeyed even in the therapeutic situation. The therapist must be flexible enough to adjust his or her style to what is called for by the client's degree of formality. The outcome of therapy depends in great part on the ability of the therapist to see beyond narrow confines of theory. The therapist has to think of the entire situation that clients might be in, and not rely solely upon what they present as their problem. If the client is ashamed, as Helena was of her children's behaviour, he or she is not likely to volunteer information. It is up to the therapist to consider what might be hidden. Therapy is a joint production and requires the therapist to pay close attention to how the client speaks, as well as to what the client is saying. This chapter concentrated on therapy with depression. The next deals with therapy for the addicted, and Chapter 5 is concerned with the far knottier problem of doing therapy with schizophrenics.

Notes

1. White H (1981) The value of narrativity in the representation of reality. In Mitchell WJT (ed) On Narrative. Chicago: University of Chicago Press, 1.
2. Labov W (1963) The social motivation of a sound change. Word 19: 273–309.
3. Giles H, Taylor D, Bourhis R (1973) Towards a theory of interpersonal accommodations through language: some Canadian data. Language

in Society 2: 177–223; Chaika E (1994) Language: The Social Mirror, 3rd edn. Boston, Mass.: Heinle & Heinle, 88–90.
4. Chaika (1994) op. cit., 81–117.
5. Erickson F (1984) Rhetoric, anecdote, and rhapsody: coherence strategies in a conversation among black American adolescents. In Tannen D (ed) Coherence in Spoken and Written Discourse, Norwood, NJ: Ablex, 81–154.
6. Baars E (1988) A Cognitive Theory of Consciousness. Cambridge: Cambridge University Press.
7. Chafe W (1994) Discourse, Consciousness, and Time. Chicago: University of Chicago Press, 53.
8. Sacks H (1992) Lectures on Conversation, Vol. 1. Jefferson G (ed). Cambridge, Mass.: Blackwell, 433.
9. Ferrara KW (1994) Therapeutic Ways with Words. New York: Oxford University Press, 71–83.
10. Gilligan C (1982) In a Different Voice: Women's Conception of Self and Morality. Cambridge, Mass.: Harvard University Press.
11. This doesn't mean that her work was faulty. It's just that scholars destruct other scholars' works. That's the way scholarship works.
12. Jack D (1991) Silencing the Self. Cambridge, Mass.: Harvard University Press, 1.
13. Ibid., 5.
14. Ibid., 8.
15. It has often struck me that this is a description of the perfect autistic or Asberger patient.
16. Ibid., 18.
17. Ibid., 7.
18. Linde C (1993) Life Stories: The Creation of Coherence. New York: Oxford University Press.
19. Jack D (1991) Silencing the Self. Cambridge, Mass.: Harvard University Press, 110.
20. Ibid., 154–68.
21. Ibid., 12.
22. Ibid., 216–18.
23. Ibid., 54.
24. Bateson G (1972) Steps to an Ecology of Mind. New York: Ballantine.
25. Jack D (1991) Silencing the Self. Cambridge, Mass.: Harvard University Press, 23–5.
26. Freyer F (1997) There's more to it than 'talk'. The Providence Sunday Journal, 26 October 1997, L2.
27. Erickson F (1984) Rhetoric, anecdote, and rhapsody: coherence strategies in a conversation among black American adolescents. In Tannen D (ed) Coherence in Spoken and Written Discourse, Norwood, NJ: Ablex, 97.
28. Erickson F, Shultz J (1982) The Counselor as Gatekeeper: Social

Interaction in Interviews. New York: Academic Press.

29. Chaika E (1994) Language: The Social Mirror, 3rd edn. Boston, Mass.: Heinle & Heinle, 162.

30. Ferrara KW (1994) Therapeutic Ways with Words. New York: Oxford University Press.

31. Ibid., 37.

32. Ferrara KW (1994) Repetition as rejoinder in therapeutic discourse: echoing and mirroring. In Johnston B (ed) Repetition in Discourse: Interdisciplinary Perspectives, Vol. 2, Advances in Discourse Processes. Norwood, NJ: Ablex, 66–83; Ferrara, Therapeutic Words, 108–27.

33. Ferrara, Therapeutic Words, 110.

34. Ibid., 11–113.

35. Ibid., 119–23.

36. Ibid., 120.

37. Ibid., 52–83.

38. Sacks H (1992) Lectures on Conversation, Vol. 1, Jefferson G (ed). Cambridge, Mass.: Blackwell, 437.

39. Such completions can also be a ploy in which one speaker wrests the floor from another. If the completion is uttered sarcastically, in a 'Yeah, I know' tone of voice, it can be even be a major put-down, of the 'You keep saying ...' type.

40. Ferrara, Therapeutic Words, 146.

41. Ibid., 152.

42. Ibid., 147.

43. Ibid., 156.

Chapter 4
Proverbs, metaphors, idioms and therapy

Strategic use of language facilitates therapeutic change.[1]

Introduction

This chapter shows the efficacy of proverbs and idioms in helping those who need to fight drug and alcohol addictions. The proverb is seen as an expression of the community, thus taking the onus of correction off the therapist. It also helps the client to feel bonded to the community. Metaphors, how they are constructed and how used in the therapeutic situation, are also explored. Metaphors are seen to be more than unusual language. One can't assume that the strange language of schizophrenics, for example, are just metaphors, for, as we see here, metaphors are created by regular processes and according to cultural models.

Proverbs

Proverbs have been shown to be extremely useful in therapy, especially in treating addictions. Like other categories in linguistics, it is not possible to draw a hard line between proverbs and similar tropes, such as slogans, idioms, or metaphor. That is, all of these have fuzzy borders, but, within these borders, there are clear instances of each. Examples of proverbs, for instance are

1. Out of sight, out of mind
2. Nothing ventured, nothing gained
3. An ounce of prevention is worth a pound of cure
4. A stitch in time saves nine
5. Absence makes the heart grow fonder
6. A rolling stone gathers no moss.

Like idioms, proverbs entail phrase structures. They may be entire sentences as in (3)–(6), but, like (1) they may just be prepositional or other phrases. (2) has an interesting structure. Strictly speaking, it is composed of two sentences. At least, each part has a subject and a predicate verb, but the first, 'Nothing ventured' is a truncated form of 'If nothing is ventured' and 'nothing gained' is a truncated 'then nothing is gained'. We expect such truncations in proverbs because, by their nature, they are supposed to be pithy. Moreover, they are supposed to be culturally familiar, and the more context a speaker shares with hearers, the fewer words that are necessary for comprehension. The ellipsis in proverbs is reminiscent of the ellipsis in ordinary conversation. Besides ellipsis, in (1)–(4), we see another common property of proverbs: parallelism. The structures within each can be divided binarily with each half structurally like the other. In (1) the prepositional *out of* is repeated. In (2), *Nothing* and the verb form are both repeated. In (3), two weights, *ounce* and *pound* are opposed to each other, each followed by the preposition *of*, and in (4) *time* and *nine* are near rhymes, a kind of parallelism. Proverbs, like poetry, also tend to have a strong stress pattern. Proverbs are also usually uttered with the voice falling at the end, as when making a definite statement. The pithiness, parallelism, stress patterns and prosody make proverbs easy to remember. All of these are mnemonic devices. The downward intonation typical of proverbs emphasizes that they are didactic. They are stating – or seem to be stating – universal verities.

One problem with this last observation is that some proverbs mean diametrically opposed things to different people or in different contexts. Honeck[2] cites the different meanings of 'A rolling stone gathers no moss'. In Scotland, it means that people should stay active. In England, it is used to tout stability, and in Texas, college students understand it to mean that one should keep moving and not be tied down by family and possessions. This is an exceptionally ambiguous proverb, however. Even so, the context in which it is delivered should usually serve to indicate which meaning the speaker intended. The meanings of (1) through (5) above, like many proverbs, are quite unambiguous even without context, although note the inconsistency between (1) and (5). But they are both true. Sometimes absence does make the heart grow fonder and sometimes out of sight, out of mind. It depends on the persons and the circumstances under which they are separating. The folk wisdom presented by proverbs takes into account the true messiness of human affairs.

Interestingly, Whaley sees the ambiguity of some proverbs as very helpful in therapy[3] because it allows for multiple meanings, so that clients may examine more than one perspective because of the 'multiple interpretations of the proverb's analogies'. Also, Whaley claims, the listener 'must decipher the proverb's connection to the conversation at hand'. Thus the ambiguity can help a therapist, especially with a client who 'has such a tight hold on a ... problem that he or she refuses to deal with anything else'. Whaley contends that if the therapist introduces ambiguity in such a situation, the client is forced to look at alternatives. I should imagine that using proverbs this way could work only if the therapist could think up an ambiguous proverb that fits the client's situation. There has to be a connection to the client. It has occurred to me, however, that at an appropriate juncture, or one in which the client finds nothing to say, the therapist could offer a proverb that fits into the client's situation and ask the client what he or she thinks the proverb means and whether or not it has relevance for the client. The next thing would be to ask how the proverb applied to the client's life, if it did at all. The client either ratifies the proverb as pertinent to his or her own life, or rejects it. In either instance, the way has been paved for more understandings and raising of new topics.

An alternative would be to mention two proverbs which contradict each other, such as 'He who hesitates is lost' versus 'Look before you leap.' The therapist can then ask the client why he or she thinks both proverbs exist side by side. What does each mean? What kinds of situations does each belong to? Perhaps 'Once bitten, twice shy' might also come up while discussing these. Again, this would be an opening for the client to relate to his or her own life.

Proverbs are typically concerned with everyday life and dilemmas. They do not refer to esoteric situations or preferences. They also tend strongly to refer to paths taken or not, or, at least, what considerations should be considered before action. Thus, as interaction openers or to jump start stalled interviews, proverbs are excellent vehicles in therapy, which itself is all about paths taken or not, or considerations before one acts. If the therapist feels that a direct question about the topic would not lead to a good discussion, or cause the client to resist or deny what needs discussing, then an appropriate proverb might get the ball rolling.[4] Proverbs are figurative enough not to be threatening. They're mundane enough so that virtually anybody can discuss their import. If anyone objects to them, it is likely to be someone who feels too intellectual for such folksy stuff, but even that person can discuss the intellectual issues raised by the proverb.

The value of a proverb sociolinguistically is that it represents the community's norms and ideals.[5] In therapy, Whaley[6] points out that reminding hearers of the proverb's community status by typical introductions like, 'You know what they say ...'

> reduces the chance that the suggestion will be seen as a personal attack and serves, instead, to attribute the recommendation to traditional wisdom. Hence, the use of some proverbs potentially removes the advice-giver's responsibility from the suggestion...

He adds that proverbs allow therapists to phrase solutions to recurring problems in an indirect, yet authoritative manner.

Whaley[7] has another interesting take on the uses of proverbs in therapy. Proverbs, he claims, are **enthymemes**. An enthymeme is a syllogism with either the premiss or the conclusion missing. For instance, one syllogism is (my example):

All canines must eat meat
Dogs are canines
Dogs must eat meat

If I said 'All dogs, being canine, must eat meat', or even 'All dogs eat meat', then, I have uttered an enthymeme, a conclusion with major or minor premisses not stated. I made the latter remark to an avid vegetarian who was keeping his dog on a vegetarian diet, expecting that the vegetarian would understand what I meant. He did, supplying both premisses, and we were able to argue the issue from there.

Whaley, using the example of 'a stitch in time saves nine' uttered to mean that cars need regular maintenance, says that a proverb, which is actually an enthymeme 'compels the receiver to provide the premise to complete the argument'.[8] Whaley feels that the therapist can then use the client's premisses 'in cooperation with the enthymemic form' to strengthen or alter problematic premisses. Unfortunately, Whaley doesn't give any examples of this being done, actually or hypothetically. He also doesn't provide the premisses that would make 'a stitch in time' a syllogism. That is, Whaley fails to show that this particular proverb is enthymatic. I must confess that I can't think of formal major and minor premisses for this particular proverb, although I see the imagery of one loose stitch causing others to come undone. Even if a proverb isn't an enthymeme, it still requires the therapist and client to work out meanings together. This fosters joint production. Also, the situation might arise in which the therapist thinks of a proverb which could be treated as an enthymeme, just as my enthymemic statement to Mr. Vegetarian happened to come up in conversation. Proverbs are good for a therapist to keep in mind, although they can't be used in all situations, nor should they be used too often. If a therapist is perceived to talk in proverbs excessively, he or she seems inflexible and, perhaps, even unimaginative. Yet, there is one situation in which much or even most of the therapy centres on proverbs and slogans: therapeutic communities devoted to breaking drug and alcohol addictions.

Therapeutic communities like Synanon and groups like Alcoholics Anonymous utilize proverbs maximally. They typically mix proverbs and slogans like 'Hang tough' and 'It's better to give than to receive' not only in talk, but in signs hung prominently in meeting areas. The proverbs and slogans remind members of their goals and expected behaviours. Since they are concise, usually have strong rhythm, and exceptional parallelism, they are also effective mnemonic devices. That is, they are easy for members to remember, and to remind themselves of their life goals even after they've left the therapeutic community.

Bassin[9] points out that when members of groups use 'proverbs, slogans, folk sayings, quotations, maxims and songs, these symbols add to the *cohesiveness of the group*' (italics his). These groups form mini-societies and, as we have seen, proverbs are folk wisdom belonging to given societies or cultural groups. As such, they are bonding devices because they make members feel that they think alike and that they share and agree upon knowledge. Proverbs and slogans make the community their reference point, offering their members a feeling of identity as part of the group. They are felt as being the norms of the group itself,[10] and by accepting and repeating them, members feel social solidarity with the others. The slogans appear 'to have an important answer to an important question' – they help communicate that the agency has the answers.[11]

Rogers[12] points out that the proverb is a genre that promotes social action. It gives advice, but it is traditional and has a social role. It takes the burden off the teller. It makes the teller a representative of the whole community, which is why proverbs are often prefaced with phrases like 'As they say ...' or 'You know what they say ...' In groups, in which members are learning to conform to a rigid set of standards in order to rid themselves of their drug and alcohol addictions, proverbs are not used to spur argumentation or self-discovery as in other kinds of therapy. Their usage is strictly traditional, to state norms which must be abided by.

It is interesting that neither Bassin nor Rogers distinguish between genres like proverbs, slogans, maxims, colloquialisms and quotations. Nor do they define them. Perhaps this is because they all have the same norma-tive function. All also have the peculiar property of usually not being questioned by the hearer. Questions can be asked of them, of course, but usually not within therapy for addictions. There, they are meant to be accepted and repeated. The difference between proverbs, slogans and quotations is largely structural.[13] We have already looked at the structure of proverbs. By their very nature, proverbs don't state things overtly. The hearer has to figure out the meaning.

In contrast, slogans typically are commands like 'Hang tough,' 'If at first you don't succeed, try, try again' or are didactic declaratives like 'No pain. No gain' or 'When the going gets tough, the tough get going.' Slogans have overt meaning and they don't usually require interpretation as proverbs do. Even those that are not in linguistic imperative form, have an implied imperative to them. For instance, 'No pain. No gain' says that you must do what is painful in order to gain a cure. And 'When the going gets tough...' indicates you have to be tough and keep with the programme, as difficult as that may be at times.

Quotations also serve the same ends as proverbs and slogans. All three belong to the community, but proverbs and slogans don't have one author, whereas quotations are attributable to sources like The Bible or to a particular person, usually a famous one. Proverbs, then, and their cousins, slogans and quotations, are of great utility in helping addicts become free of their habits. Here they serve to remind and reinforce. They are meant to be repeated and their meaning is limited. In other kinds of therapy, discussing the meaning of tropes is a way to spur discussion. So, the same vehicle, proverbs, can be utilized beneficially in diametrically opposed ways.

Metaphor

Metaphor figures largely in the literature of psychotherapy and in the literature on understanding schizophrenia. Because metaphor-making and metaphorical boundaries of meaning are so often misunderstood, it is important to consider what metaphors actually are and how they are created, before discussing their uses in therapy.

Language is suffused with metaphor. We hear and use metaphors constantly, but are often unaware of them. Beck[14] points out that 'one of the most exciting and overall attributes to human thought' is its ability to enlarge its grasp on to problems through metaphor. Beck also asserts that metaphoric reasoning is a skill independent of what we usually measure as 'intelligence'. When we think of metaphor, we naively think of literature and poetry, not everyday language. Yet, metaphor is a common, everyday way of making the words in our mental lexicons take on new meanings. When Thomas Edison first invented the electric light bulb, it is doubtful that it even occurred to many people that a new metaphor had been created. Up to that time, *bulb* referred to a kind of subterranean fleshy globe which produces plants like daffodils. Earlier, *bulb* meant 'onion,' so its meaning for flowers was originally a metaphoric extension. Edison's bulb was even more of an extension. Now the bulb was no longer vegetation, but it was round and rays of light emanated from it as leaves do from the plant bulb. The visual similarity between the old and new meanings of *bulb* is typical of metaphor, and so was Edison's practice of making old language do new duty.

Similarly, a *dial* was first a round object which showed the time divisions of a day. Then it came to refer to any round object with numbers or other markings on it to show measurement. The telephone in its first stage required people to call an operator to get connected to another phone, so you had to *ring* someone up by turning the telephone crank and having the operator cause a bell to ring at the phone you wanted to be attached to. This usage has remained alive. After this first stage, the rotary with fingerholes and numbers under it was quickly called *dial*. From this emanated the verb *dial* as in 'dial the number.' When touchtone phones came out, they had a square section of push buttons, but this array was also called a dial, despite the mismatch of shape to the original dial. The verb *to dial* remained as well although there was no longer a dial to dial, and kinetically, dialling is quite different from pushing buttons. Often part of the meaning of a word is the action associated with it, but function is also a part of a word's meaning. With the rotary phone, there was a visual similarity to the original *sundial*, but the connection with a touchtone dial is purely that of function. Both visual and functional similarities can figure in metaphor.

I stress that metaphor is actually everyday stuff because so many people have operated under the impression that it is unusual and associated with artistic uses of language. Since many artistic metaphors are difficult to understand and often require the interpretation of an expert, such as a poetry professor, some also assume that any unusual, not easily decipherable word usages are metaphorical; hence, the belief of some psychiatrists that schizophrenic speech is metaphorical because it is so difficult to understand.

Much has also been made of the fact that metaphor is a change of meaning and requires special cognitive skills. Catherine Sullivan,[15] for instance, claims that since a metaphorical usage involves changing, using metaphors helps patients to change their mind-sets. One problem with such a view is that people create and understand metaphors regularly in ordinary speech, advertising, and in literature and it doesn't necessarily make them change *their* mind sets in any way. Before discussing this, however, let us consider some other facets of word meaning.

As we saw in Chapter 1, all words are polysemous and can be used in a variety of situations. Their actual meaning is derived from the context in which they are used. This applies equally to metaphor. Both *bulb* and *dial*, for instance, are still used in their original meanings. Many scholars and practitioners think that a given metaphor may have a virtually unlimited number of meanings. Because metaphors do not show a direct link to their meaning, they think a metaphor can mean anything the reader's ingenuity can force it to mean. We see this when therapists assign a global meaning to a schizophrenic utterance, calling any strange or deviant utterance a metaphor, then assigning it a global meaning, taking little or no notice of actual words used, as in David Forrest's interpretation shown below. However, metaphors have definite derivable meanings. Each metaphor is strongly constrained by context. They are also constrained by the literal meanings of the words used in the metaphor.

As noted above, some therapists,[16] not realizing that metaphor is structured language intended to provide a particular meaning, assume that all deviant schizophrenic productions are simply unusual metaphors. Such therapists don't – and can't – justify how they derived their meaning other than saying 'It's metaphorical'. However, as we shall now see, metaphors are not deviant language and their meaning can be derived by usual means of decoding. If lexical items could take on any meaning an interpreter wishes to give them, then they would actually have no meaning. A lexical item, metaphor included, has meaning only because it has at least one semantic feature pertinent to the context. Which feature one is to catch in order to understand is usually limited by what the context allows. It is for this reason that I reject the notion that the bizarre word salads of schizophrenics, for instance, are metaphorical. They illustrate speech out of control – and in metaphor, speech is very much in control.

Within a culture, certain words have direct metaphorical meaning, such as, in English, calling someone *honey* or *sugar*, or calling someone a *dog* or a *pussy cat*. Metaphor is not merely unusual usage of a word or phrase. There has to be some kind of relationship between the metaphor and more literal words for what is meant. I can tell you 'My husband is a teddy bear' and you get an image of him as a cuddly, easy-going, loving male, but if I tell you 'My husband is a purple balloon flower' I have simply said something bizarre, unless, of course, I have managed to give enough context so that some meaning can be derived from that.

Some people define metaphors as similes without the *like* or *as*, citing examples like 'My husband is like a teddy-bear' as meaning the same thing as 'My husband is a teddy-bear.' Two or more tropes, like two or more literal words may mean the same thing in certain contexts, but, still, metaphors and similes are not identical. Consider the metaphor 'She's a peach' as opposed to the simile 'She's like a peach.' The metaphor, a frozen one, means she's sweet and good, an easy going and good-natured person. The simile yields a different reaction. Eight out of the ten people I tried it out on got no meaning from it at all, and the other two got negative meanings. One thought it meant that she's soft and plump, not firm. The other posited that she bruises easily like a peach. Another example would be 'My new car is a lemon,' which does not have a counterpart simile 'My new car is like a lemon'.

So, some words can be used to give a metaphorical meaning, but similes using the same word yield another meaning or no meaning at all. Besides this difference between metaphor and simile, there is a difference in functional usages between many metaphors and similes using the same word. In conversation, for instance, the simile is often used when the speaker wants to give a lengthier explanation. If I say 'Susie is a doll,' I am merely describing her metaphorically, but if I say, 'Susie is like a doll,' the hearer is waiting to hear why I labelled her this way. Normally the simile would be continued, as in 'Susie is like a doll. She never has a thought of her own. She just sits around and looks pretty.' Note that this is quite a different meaning from the metaphor 'Susie is a doll' which means that Susie is a good-natured person, often one who is generous with her time and who helps out willingly. One can add information to a metaphor if one wants to, but a metaphor doesn't promise the kind of extension that a simile does.

Another reason not to confuse similes with metaphors is that metaphors can be verbs as well as nouns, but similes can't. For instance, when we say 'They were *nosing* around,' the verb *nosing* is a metaphor. Metaphors can also be adjectives as in, 'They sure were *nosy*.' These may not be the best examples because the use of *nose* as a verb and adjective has become so common that it may have crossed the line into literal language for many speakers. The original image of a dog, for instance, sniffing his surroundings may be lost to them. A person's snooping was compared to a dog's poking his nose into nooks and crannies to smell information. Much of our common vocabulary is suffused with verbalizations that were once metaphorical, such as 'the *legs* of the table', 'the *foot* of the bed' and 'he *goes*' to mean 'he says' or 'he *rambled* all over *the place*' when speaking of someone speaking with no discernible purpose. Such metaphors exist in all languages and are a natural outcome of the human ability to extend the meanings of words, either because a new term is needed to refer to a new object or activity, or because a more colourful term is wanted. Metaphors enable us to express new messages using our old language as well as to say the same old thing in a less boring way. It is part of our being human to appreciate creativity in language. Metaphor is an ordinary language function with its own rules and conditions for creation and comprehension.

Some metaphors have cultural or mythological stereotypes as part of their meanings. For instance 'Man is a wolf' never means for us that 'man is monogamous, loves his offspring, and cares for them'. Yet, wolves are highly monogamous, and the male does help care for and feed his young. The metaphorical value of *wolf*, however, always refers to its predatory characteristics which fit into our cultural mythology of wolves being dangerous killers. Also, although wolves are monogamous, in older American slang a male called 'a wolf' referred to a man who tried to get many women to date him. That is, he preyed on women. As with our current usage, the image of a wolf preying informed this metaphor. Even in the word *werewolf*, we see the image of wolf as bloody, dangerous predator. The only non-mythological metaphor for *wolf* that I can see is in reference to eating. 'He wolfed his food down.' The imagery here is the fact that wolves (and dogs, who are simply domesticated wolves) eat rapidly, tearing off large chunks of meat at a time.

Beck[17] sees uncontrolled free association as the heart of human creativity and metaphor in language. She uses as her example

> Ask me where an apple comes from and I will instantly picture a supermarket, my apple tree, a seed, a Linaenian diagram, plus Adam and Eve …

She says that a critic would say that free association is not a metaphor, but she retorts that the hallmark of human intelligence and creativity is precisely the mental slipping around 'between verbal and nonverbal, part and whole, process and structure, feeling and logic' and that this is so fast that often she can't hold any single perspective responsible for a specific outcome. She then goes on to ask

> What about my association of apples with the 'Apple' computer company, and its recent product, the Macintosh? How did a computer firm come to call itself 'Apple?'

The kind of uncontrolled rapid free associating she describes sounds like what schizophrenics do,[18] and it is a bar to thought. It certainly doesn't produce intellectual or even artistic works. It certainly does not capture the careful connection between a metaphorical meaning of a word and a more literal word. Actually, although it may have been below the level of consciousness, calling a computer 'Apple' was a very controlled process. In our culture, we know that the apple Eve ate represented knowledge. Computers are used for scholarly and business knowledge. They are 'intelligent' machines, so Apple is a particularly apt name for them. A Macintosh is a popular kind of apple; hence, its use as the name for the Apple computer. One may have come to this by free-associating with the word *apple* as Beck says, but why would Apple's founder have started free-associating to come up with the name of his computer? Rather, he made a direct cultural connection between his intelligent, knowledgeable machines and a symbol for knowledge, the apple. In fact, far from being products of random associations, metaphors form tightly knit sets and rest upon firm, culturally based cognitive structures.

Often, people think of metaphor as being rooted in deviance and as calling for special construal. Certainly, such a view has been widely held in psychotherapy. Frequently, this has paved the way for highly ingenious interpretations which have no bearing on the actual words used. For instance, David Forrest[19] interprets as metaphorical

> Doctor, I have pains in my chest and hope and wonder if my box is broken and heart is beaten for my soul and salvation and heaven, Amen.

Forrest says, 'The listener is told if he has ears for it what it is like to be schizophrenic ..., but as no one who is not schizophrenic can fully empathize with this experience, the message is redirected to God's ear.' Notice there are no words or phrases in the above which convey what Forrest says it does. He is giving a global interpretation to the entire utterance. Maher,[20] on the other hand, interprets this as the patient's complaint in 'the shattered language of schizophrenia' about physical chest pains which could indicate a fatal heart condition. The question is whether this passage is metaphorical or is it intended as a literal message, one that has gone wrong because of a speech dysfunction? If we see metaphor as random deviations that allow us to suspend our usual strategies for understanding, then Forrest's interpretation is viable, but if we recognize metaphor as being controlled and rational, following definite rules for creation, then Maher is correct. Maher – rightly, I think–says this passage means that the patient is having chest pains and is worried about his heart. The rest of this utterance 'and soul and salvation and heaven' is the sort of chaining of words related either phonologically or semantically, or both, which is a characteristic of schizophrenic speech (Chapter 5). This chain may have been triggered by the speaker's fear of death from a heart attack.

One way to resolve this issue is to compare the above with passages presented by Hallowell and Smith[21] in which a schizophrenic patient whose speech was under control describes his illness as making him a prisoner, then speaks of ebbing sand below him, and of plummeting downward towards corrosive and sharp knife-like objects, such as acid, spikes, cobra spears, 'tigerhunting forks' and numerous blades. The vivid imagery of ground that is not firm and items which give horrendous pain seems to me to be a description of what it is like to be schizophrenic. Those of us who have never had the experience of being schizophrenic certainly can feel the horror that this patient is going through. But notice, the metaphors for the illness are not random. They are not just unusual usages of words. Rather, they all evoke imagery of unpredictability (ebbing sands), or sharp, cutting and biting pain. They fit together into a cohesive whole. We can analyse the metaphors by comparing them with literal words for the same ideas, and we easily see how the parts fit into a whole, creating a message.

Literary scholars also have thought of metaphor as deviant usages allowing creative interpretations. Samuel Levin[22] gives as an example of deviant usage, one which calls for special decodings the term *devouring books*, in which a term for eating transfers to reading. Actually, there is an entire set of metaphors correlating cognitive and gustatory ingestion and excretion: *juicy story, food for thought, consuming knowledge, gulping down facts, digesting information, letting ideas cook, internalize knowledge, soaking up facts, indigestible news, regurgitating facts, spilled the beans, starved for knowledge, eating it up,*[23] *spit it out, gushed forth, spewing words,* and *sharing knowledge.* Far from being deviant, we see a metaphor like *devouring books* as part of a cognitive image in which knowledge, like food, is assumed to enter the body, adding to whatever is already there. Eventually this knowledge, also like food, may exit the body as well. If it exits when it shouldn't, in English, rather unpleasant metaphors evocative of spitting or vomiting are employed. It's interesting to see that words for culturally impolite or disgusting emissions of body fluids are used to indicate that someone is displaying knowledge that he or she is supposed to be quiet about. This rounds out our cognitive model for knowledge. However, we can also share knowledge, which is also a way of letting it out, but one which evokes a pleasant and socially responsible act, just as we share food or other material goods. The very fact that we can find so many metaphors analogous to Levin's indicates that we are dealing with normal aspects of language, not deviant usages. In fact, we see a discernible cognitive model underlying English metaphors and idioms for learning: that the body is a container which fills up with knowledge, which is food. This cognitive model of the body as a container which can be filled or emptied underlies other sets of metaphors as well.

This is confirmed by several studies, notably Lakoff and Johnson,[24] Lakoff,[25] and Lakoff and Turner,[26] which have dissected several sets of metaphors, showing that metaphor making is not random creativity. They show that metaphors refer to cognition, that there is 'a coherent conceptual organization underlying' metaphorical expression.[27] Metaphors for anger, for instance, relate to the actual physiological changes wrought by anger: agitation, increased body temperature, increased blood pressure, redness in the face, and interference with accurate perception. As with the set of knowledge metaphors, those for anger are based upon a model of the body as a container, in this instance, for emotions. The body as container gets filled up, this time with a fluid. Note that most metaphors for knowledge visualize that as being solid. Anger itself is metaphorically a fluid which rises as the anger grows. At first blush it might seem that metaphors for anger are disparate metaphors, but looking at them as being constructed on a cognitive model reveals how they are related. Examples of these are:

1. get hopping mad
2. shaking with anger
3. get hot under the collar
4. a heated argument
5. blood was boiling
6. reach the boiling point
7. let him/her stew
8. burst a blood vessel
9. face red with anger
10. blind with rage
11. so mad he/she couldn't see straight.

There are even metaphors for extreme anger which refer to exploding, a combination of heat, agitation, and pressure rising to the point of explosion, as in

12. vent anger
13. letting off steam
14. flipped his/her lid
15. blew his/her stack
16. hit the ceiling
17. went through the roof.

Lakoff observes that certain otherwise inexplicable idioms for anger are actually caused by these physiologically based metaphors. For instance, expressions like 'she had kittens when I told her' are based upon the model of 'something that was inside causing pressure bursts out'. This is related to metaphors like (12)–(14) above. In (13) the fluid gets so hot, it turns to steam. This is a reference to boiling. Interestingly all these metaphors for anger work only for humans, although other animals get enraged. Some, like 'flipping one's lid' or 'blowing one's stack' depend upon an image of a creature which is two-legged and stands erect, so that their 'lid' is where the lid on a jar is, on top, like a human head. Similarly 'stack' elicits an image of upright, bipedal stance. In *More than Cool Reason*, Lakoff and Turner show that underlying cognitive models for other matters like life, death, and time have remained consistent for centuries, as evidenced in poetry from Chaucer to today.

This doesn't mean that someone can't make up a metaphor that doesn't conform to these models. They can, but certain constraints do exist. For instance, we have seen three important factors underlying metaphor. The first is our shared cultural knowledge, as in the naming of the Apple computer. The second is our awareness of our own physiological states, such as feeling hot, or getting red-faced when angry. The third is visual. Metaphors are often vivid pictures. Note the imagery in devouring a book or hitting the ceiling. Even single non-metaphorical words may be based upon visual imagery. Words denoting stinginess, for instance, often invoke a picture of grasping tightly to one's body, so that a stingy person can be said to be 'tightfisted'. This conforms to the reality, that a stingy person is someone who holds on to things. Our visual image of this is one of keeping the fingers closed and the arms close to the body. Any new word we make up to indicate miserliness conforms to this visual imagery. We couldn't decide to call a miser 'openfingered', but we could call him 'tightfingered' or 'closehanded', both of which retain the imagery of a grasping person. I recently heard someone described as 'hugging' his possessions which not only accords with the visual of holding something closely, not letting it go, but also indicates the degree of his fondness for his things.

Metaphors may also be formed by collocating words in an unusual manner, just so long as the context makes them decipherable. Additionally, once a hearer recognizes that a statement must be metaphorical, he or she calls upon principles of decoding which are applied to the metaphor in order to get its meaning. These principles involve a general strategy of 'What can this possibly mean here?' at the same time ignoring the inherent semantic features not germane to the context. Gibbs[28] gives as examples *These tires are my vacation* and *This room is a toilet*. The former meant 'because I had to buy these tires, I can't afford to go on a vacation.' Culturally, we know that buying tires does not fit into our cognitive model of what a vacation is, so we hear the metaphor as either a joke or a complaint, or both. The second example, unless said while pointing out the loo, was not literally a toilet. The room mentioned was just very dirty. Gibbs also mentions as a metaphor ...*Willie Nelson has more music in the oven* ... We can understand this because we know if food is in the oven, it is being prepared for consumption, but music in the oven must mean music that is in the process of being composed. This is reminiscent of the way we speak of ideas 'cooking', so a cognitive model has been tapped into, that of food preparation and products of our intelligence.

This is a subdivision of the cognitive model which equates learning with eating.

Suppose one's friend said, 'Oh, you can't come over right now. This place is a pigsty.' One property of a pigsty is that it is used to house four-legged non-human pigs. Since it is not likely that the room is literally a pigsty, then the speaker must intend that the hearer take a property of *pigsty* and apply it to her room. Pigsties are dirty and odoriferous, so, metaphorically, the speaker means that the room is a mess. For emphasis, we often use **hyperbole** as well, exaggeration, so the hearer assumes that the room may be messy and dirty, but probably not as dirty and odoriferous as a real pigsty. Another example is someone who says 'Movies are my life.' Obviously nobody's entire life is movies. One must eat and sleep and perhaps even go to work. Usually one has some friends, colleagues, spouses, children or other kin to interact with. Consequently, the hearer interprets this as hyperbole as well as metaphor, meaning that the speaker is an avid movie buff, probably knows a great deal about them, possibly has taken formal film courses, reads a lot about them, knows who starred in what, who various directors were and what movies they made, and so on.

We can fashion a multitude of utterances on these two models alone, further showing how usual such metaphoric statements are: my room is a **palace**, that is a **den** of iniquity, my house is a **jewel**, my husband is a **pussy-cat**, my car is a **lemon**; my children are my **life**, **my diamond ring** is my son's college education ... Metaphors are not confined to these sentence patterns. They can occur as nouns, verbs, or adjectives in any utterance type, but the general principles are the same, both of encoding and decoding.

Other explanations for figurative language, such as Weinreich's (1966) presentation of the role of semantic features in meaning also point to the regularity of metaphorical processes. One of his examples was *pretty boy* which achieves its meaning of a less than masculine male by transferring the feature of [+feminine] which inheres in *pretty* onto *boy*. Weinreich thought that adjectives always transfer features on to nouns, but Adrienne Lehrer[29] in her study of the semantics of wine testing, shows that transfer can go from the noun to the adjective. For instance, in *velvety wine* it is the word *wine* which tells us which semantic feature(s) of *velvet* we should take for its meaning. The inherent meaning of velvet, cloth with a nap on it, cannot be used. Literally, wine like velvet would be disgusting. The mouth feel would be gagging. In her study of terms for wine, Lehrer had people at a wine-tasting describe the flavour of wines. They used terms like *oaky*, *lamb*, and even *burning leaves* as in the fall, to describe the wines. Interestingly, in light of what we've stressed about achieving bonding in therapeutic sessions, Lehrer found that when subjects first disagreed in the meanings of the words they used to describe wine, they would discuss their choices until they came to an agreement. They reported feeling rapport after successfully negotiating meaning.

George Miller[30] shows how deixis, actually pointing to something, which is usually considered to be straightforward and literal, can also be metaphorical. For instance, in a restaurant, a waiter can point to a ham sandwich and say 'the man in red' to mean 'he ordered it' or 'bring it to him'. Similar usages occur with 'the hot fudge sundae practically licked the plate clean' meaning 'the person who ordered the hot fudge sundae ...' There is an added visually based metaphor here, that of a dog or other animal who licks its plate. Metaphor suffuses every aspect of language and any utterance can contain several. Outside of a first grade reading primer like *Dick and Jane*, it is hard to find speech which is not infused with metaphor.

Many, if not most, metaphors are single words, as when we speak of the *underpinnings* of a theory, a *tidal wave* of feeling, behaving *coldly*, or *heated* discussions. These words can also be used literally in different contexts. For instance, the word *heated* means quite different things in 'a heated discussion' and 'heated soup'. Context tells us when a word is being used metaphorically. If I say that my human friend Otis devours books, I mean he's an avid reader, but I can also say that my dog Otis devours books and I mean that he really chews them up and swallows them.

Sternberg, Torangeau, and Nigro,[31] in their discussion of metaphor creation, themselves use a metaphor of meaning based upon associations with a rubber band. Sternberg et al. point out that one can *stretch* a meaning of a word only up to a point, and then it *snaps* (pp. 334–5). The very metaphor they use to delineate the limits of metaphor seems to be one of those physiologically based metaphors which Lakoff and Johnson so aptly showed to be at the foundation of human metaphorizing. We bend and stretch our bodies such as stretching to reach something or bending to fit under something, so the metaphor has an origin in human physiology. These metaphors also show the role that the function and properties of an item have in our being able to create metaphors. Rubber bands are typically stretched to fit over the items one wants to hold together, and they also can conform to many shapes. Metaphorically, then, meaning is *elastic*, we *stretch the truth*, we *bend the meaning* to our purpose, meaning is *flexible*. All of these are based upon the tactile and visual experience of bending and stretching materials to fit a purpose.

Sometimes a dialectal difference will yield a different aesthetic to a metaphor. In my dialect, for instance, *elastic* is the term for 'rubber band', so that 'meaning is elastic' is vividly metaphorical, and immediately calls up the entire set of meaning: snapping, being stretchable and flexible. Although the metaphors may be based on properties of what other dialects call a *rubber band*, notice that *rubber band* is itself not metaphorical. 'Meaning is a rubber band' has no metaphorical value, at least for me, although the simile 'meaning is like a rubber band' can work figuratively, but not as well as *elastic*.[32]

Sternberg et al. make an important point, which is that there are limits to metaphorical meaning. One can't take a word and use it to mean whatever one's ingenuity and fancy come up with. The metaphorical meaning arises from the literal one and the metaphorical has to have a connection with the literal. The hearer has to be able to expand the meaning of the word(s) used. It is part of our normal linguistic baggage both as speakers and listeners that we recognize when the extension has snapped. This is why we hear disordered schizophrenic speech as deviant, not metaphorical.

One has to question seriously interpretations so *strained* (another metaphor of the *elastic* set) that normal decodings, even normal informed decodings, cannot be traced to the words that were actually employed. Decodings of metaphor have to be based upon the semantic features of those words, as well as the visual and physiological imagery demanded by the words being interpreted. If the metaphor belongs to a set, like those for *anger* above, then it often conforms to the underlying cognitive models.

This doesn't mean that novel metaphors can't be created or interpreted. Obviously, they can. Also, not all metaphors inhere in sets with underlying cognitive models. Metaphors can be created by forcing (metaphorically speaking) hearers to take two or more words that aren't in the same domain or do not ordinarily collocate with each other, and then make sense of them because a sensory or functional similarity can be evoked, as in Dylan Thomas's 'the sweethearting crib', Richard Wilbur's 'a giant absence', or Emily Dickinson's 'furnished souls'. The essence of wit, of comedy, of drama, of the verbal arts in all their forms all depend upon novel metaphorizing. Usually, we perceive metaphorical meaning with no trouble. As we've seen, metaphors abound in every day speech.[33] All explanations for metaphorical meaning must be based upon the kinds of extensions of meaning discussed here and must conform to what we know about metaphors. They are word based. They are context based. Most important, one can't claim a meaning for an entire discourse without referring it to all its parts. By 'all its parts', I don't mean necessarily just individual words. Sometimes phrases get used as single units of meaning, especially in idioms, which are discussed in the next section.

Rumelhart[34] claims that the same comprehension strategies are used in interpreting figurative language as literal because the studies he cites show that that it takes no longer to assign a figurative meaning to a sentence in context than it does to assign a non-figurative one. What does take longer is assigning a meaning to a sentence out of context. Clark and Lucy[35] found that it took only about 0.3 seconds longer to comprehend a request in figurative language than a literal one.

Beck[36] found that other studies have shown that the meaning of metaphor is often grasped more rapidly than literal speech encoding the same thought. Memory tests have also shown that people remember and retain metaphoric encodings as easily as literal ones. Studies have also shown that verbal material with high image rating is easier to recall than that with lower image rating, and metaphors typically are highly imagistic. When we combine this finding with studies that show that more recall occurs with highly structured material than with less structured, we realize the degree to which metaphor itself is structured. If it weren't, people wouldn't be able to comprehend and remember metaphors so well.

We've already seen that the context-bound nature of language is well-known, and applies to metaphorical as well as literal meanings. All linguistic constructions ultimately mean what the context allows them to mean. For this reason, we can use phrases that are patently untrue, as in metaphor, but still manage to convey a real meaning. I would go one step further and point out that metaphor is possible only because of the context-dependency of language and its lack of isomorphism between message and meaning. Since there is no necessary one-to-one correspondence between linguistic structures and what they signify, we can, within constraints, extend lexical items to create new meanings or to repeat old ones in a novel way.

A distinction is commonly made between 'dead' and 'live' metaphors, with expressions like *the heart of the matter* being recognized as having their origin in metaphor, but which are now so common that they are virtually literal. In practice, it is frequently difficult to delineate a sharp boundary between dead and live metaphors. Virtually any non-concrete word can be seen to have as its origin a concrete one. It must be that human language started out with words only for the palpable, the visible and the smellable. By extension, these became used in different domains and some became more and more abstract. Saying that a clock has a *face* is a transfer from one domain to another. Speaking of *face* value makes the word more abstract. It is impossible to conceive of a word so concrete or so frequently used as a metaphor that it couldn't be used anew metaphorically. Somebody might even find a new way to use *heart* in yet another metaphorical sense. In therapy, then, we should expect both therapist and client to use metaphor. Before discussing the uses of metaphor in therapy, let us briefly look at the differences and similarities between metaphors and idioms.

Idioms

Idioms are grammatically correct linguistic structures consisting of syntactic phrases, such as prepositional phrases, or even entire predicates. Typically, subjects have to be combined with the idiom to create a complete sentence or utterance. Idioms, however, act like single words in that the idiomatic portion of the sentence typically can be paraphrased by one word, either a literal or a metaphorical one. The idiomatic phrase is an oddity in language in that it is typically limited to one meaning, often replaceable by one word. Given the polysemy and polyfunction of most linguistic structures, idioms are oddities, but bountiful ones. You can't derive the meaning of an idiom by dissecting its words and phrase structure. However, you can explain some idioms in terms of the cognitive structures mentioned above or by relating them to known historical facts. Others are explicable by their visual imagery alone. Many metaphors are also idioms, although not all idioms are metaphors. For instance, 'blew his/her stack' is a metaphorical idiom conforming to the image of heated pressure building up causing an explosion with *stack* as a metaphor for a person's body. The body is a stack, the top of which can blow off. It is also an idiom in that it is a phrase which has to be taken together to equal one word, here 'exploded'. Idioms are usually highly visual, and portray vivid pictures, as in the following:

1.	upset the apple cart	'disturb'
2.	be over the hill	'get old'
3.	sell X down the river	'betray'
4.	pull X's leg	'tease'
5.	bought the farm	'died'
6.	gone to the other side	'died'
7.	hanging by a thread	'precarious'
8.	shake the dew off the lily	'urinate'
9.	worship the porcelain god	'vomit'
10.	shoot the breeze	'chat'

Notice that these belong to the more casual registers of language. Typically, taboo subjects like death, urinating and vomiting elicit idioms in speakers, perhaps because the idiom is such a roundabout way of expressing these. The other topics of idioms are mundane, but the idiom is more colourful than a literal word would be. Upsetting the applecart evokes a vivid picture of the overturned cart with apples rolling every which way and an agitated vendor. Both (3) and (5) refer to historical incidents in America, although I have heard many British speakers use them as well.

Idioms are different from proverbs in that they are almost never in the form of complete sentences[37] and are not didactic. They don't have the parallelism of proverbs either, and proverbs usually aren't replaceable by one word as idioms are. Proverbs also often have more than one possible meaning. Idioms don't. Although idioms and metaphors overlap, idioms are different from most metaphors in that their meaning is frozen and they can't be put into new collocations. In contrast, virtually any word used in a new, but comprehensible way can be given a metaphorical meaning. One example is Emily Dickinson's collocating *furnished* with *souls* in her poem 'Cambridge Ladies with Furnished Souls'. Any interpretation of this metaphor, like all metaphors, must consider the literal meanings of both *furnished* and *soul*. For instance, one can't decide that this means that Cambridge ladies are rich monetarily or that they are open-minded. A furnished soul is one that is no longer amenable to growth. It is filled with hard ideas. These ladies are smug. One may disagree with my interpretation, but that disagreement must take into account both words in their usual literal meanings, and then see which parts of the meanings of each word can be combined to make sense. In this case, the meaning has to fit the rest of the poem as its context. The rest of the poem makes it clear that these are smug, narrow-minded women. In what follows, we must remember, however, that most metaphors aren't this esoteric. Ordinary language is suffused with them. Metaphors overlap with idioms which, virtually by definition, belong to ordinary speech.

Metaphors and therapy

Early on, those working with the mentally ill have been concerned with metaphor. Like David Forrest, noting that psychotic patients often used strange, even bizarre language, they assumed the language was metaphorical. Metaphors, however, are not simply strange and bizarre language, as we have seen. They are not randomly produced and they do have specific meanings.

Pollio et al.[38] show that therapists frequently use the client's metaphors more often than they use the ones they themselves initiated. In their study, 16 out of 26 metaphors therapists used were originally patient-initiated and only five were originally therapist-initiated. Unfortunately, Pollio et al. do not give any of the actual metaphors used by either group, nor do they provide sample interviews. Presuming their data are accurate, we see that their findings indicate that the alert therapist does pick up on his or her clients' words and uses them to further therapy. It also shows the frequency of metaphor in therapeutic situations and how natural it is for clients to express themselves metaphorically.

Several researchers and therapists have posited that metaphor can be useful in therapy. Catherine Sullivan,[39] for instance, extrapolates from the fact that metaphor involves a change in usual meaning that 'the utterance of a metaphor implicitly necessitates a change. Furthermore, this change presents a shift in interpretation by the participants.' She prefaces this statement by claiming that the structure of metaphor brings with it a change such that the standard meaning of one word or phrase is changed by the juxtaposition with another word or phrase. By this criterion, every lexical item in the language is a metaphor and virtually every phrase is one, because all words are polysemous, and all derive their meaning partially by the other words they are juxtaposed to. Sullivan[40] claims that

> the patient is locked into one world view ... with no apparent way out. The
> metaphor allows the patient to transcend that context through reference to

> another context ...This simultaneously reveals to the patient his or her capacity
> to shift out of a context, which previously was thought to be immutable.

She is correct that patients are often locked into one world view, but that doesn't mean that hearing a metaphor will show them that they are so confined and need to change. In other words, Sullivan claims that because metaphors take a word from one domain and extend it to another, they cause hearers to see that change is possible. From what has already been shown about metaphors above, we see the fallacies inherent in this view. First, we have seen that everyday language is loaded with metaphors, dead, alive and moribund. Do hearers note all the metaphors they hear? They can't all cause people to 'shift out of a context' and if they did everyone would be in a constant flux. People would never have to complain about 'being in a rut'! Another problem with Sullivan's view is that, in any given stretch of language, different people will identify different expressions as metaphoric. Do you count 'legs of the chair' as a metaphor? Once it was, but does the hearer today perceive the mapping from the domains of animals to that of furniture? 'How about 'stars in her eyes?' Is *stars* here still a metaphor? Do hearers note that *stars* have crossed domains? And if they do, how will this help get them to change their way of thinking?

Usually, as shown above, metaphors are decoded as rapidly as literal language and by using the same methods of decoding as are used for literal language: matching words to context, including what other words have been said, and then figuring which of the many semantic features attached to each word will blend with the context. This indicates that people do not go through an added step of figuring out the original domain of a metaphor and how it was mapped on to a new one. In fact, Sullivan offers no corroborating data to show how often someone actually recognizes or consciously notes what metaphors another is using. It is probable that, given the same segment of speech, people will not all mark the same words or phrases as being metaphorical. What is a dead metaphor to me, may be moribund to you, and still alive to someone else.

Taken literally, Sullivan's stance is not viable. However, she is not entirely wrong. Good, vivid or witty figurative language can keep someone interested in the therapeutic situation, and therapy can change lives. In a laboratory situation, subjects do remember vivid expressions better than non-vivid ones, but there is no evidence that this effects behavioural change directly. It's what message is encoded in the figurative language, and the discussions that ensue from it, that sometimes change behaviour.

If hearing a metaphor is persuasive, it is because the content of the metaphor, or, more usually, of the entire argument, is persuasive. If we keep repeating the same messages in the same wordings, then we are harping on things. We are nags. We are bores. Metaphors and other figurative language allow us to say old things in a myriad of new ways and, linguistic creatures that we are, we enjoy the word play, the unusualness of new encodings. Figurative language of all kinds, witticisms and jokes make repetitions more palatable, so they might not be tuned out, but it's the message behind the figurative language that is then noted, not the fact that domains have been crossed. Unfortunately, even if someone gets the message, it doesn't necessarily effect change. If it did, then raising children wouldn't be so hard, and being a parent, a teacher, scholar, clergyman or psychotherapist wouldn't be such a study in frustration.

Sullivan[41] demonstrates, quoting from one of Erickson's therapy sessions which utilized an extended metaphor. She sees metaphor in highly vivid terms, quoting Turner,[42] that metaphor allows components of one system [to] enter into **dynamic** (emphasis mine) relations with components of the other. She also claims that Erickson exploits the dynamic interaction between the elements to effect behavioural change.

She gives as an example Erickson's intended equation between dining habits and a couple's sexual relations. In this, Erickson never mentions sex at all. Rather, he presents to his clients how couples may be mismatched in their dining habits, the wife likes appetizers, whereas the husband wants to dive right into the main course, or the wife wants the dinner to be leisurely, but the husband wants to get it over with. If the couple seemed to start to make a connection with sex in all this dinner talk, Erickson does not ratify their understanding. Rather, he just changes the topic, but at the end of the session, he advises them to have dinner on a particular evening. There is no mention of any post-session contact which could verify that the couple understood that Erickson was really talking about sexual styles. At one point, he thought they might have, but his response to that was an immediate change of direction. It seems to me that if the couple thought they understood his metaphor, they might interpret his change of topic as meaning they did not understand it and they could be left drifting in the sea.[43] As part of his therapeutic methodology, he refuses to translate. Even if the couple did understand his point, there are no follow-up data that prove that they did have sex on that night or that their sex lives had been improved. There certainly was no comparison with couples who went to sex counsellors who give overt techniques and behaviours to follow to improve couples' sex lives, although this would confirm or disconfirm whether metaphor is superior for effecting change than literal language is, at least for this purpose.

There is one other thing militating against Erickson's using dining out as a metaphor for sex unless he expressly connected the metaphor of sex to eating. Our cognitive models for metaphors of passion are not primarily about food. Recall that we do use food imagery to represent knowledge metaphorically, but for sex, most of our metaphors are those of heat, non-human animals, and the use of male carpentering tools. This last fulfils the conditions for an underlying cognitive model of sex.

1. To have the hots for X.
2. X has hot pants.
3. You light my fire.
4. She's a hottie.
5. You bring out the beast in me ... (said admiringly).
6. She's a tigress.
7. She's like a bitch in heat.
8. What a stud.
9. He hammered her.
10. He screwed her.
11. He banged her.
12. He nailed her.
13. What an animal (said admiringly).

(9)–(13) represent an unfortunate cognitive model of the female being worked on violently by the male. The numbers of rapes and assaults on women in our society indicate that, too often, this is how some men perceive sex and females. As for food imagery, we do have:

14. He's sex-starved.
15. I hunger for your touch.

Older slang also had:

16. What a dish
17. She's a real tomato

but these are moribund in usage. My students get no sexual connotations for them at all, and, unlike (1)–(13), they express admiration, but don't necessarily have an association with the sex act itself.

We have, more neutrally, the non-metaphorical euphemisms 'making love', 'going to bed with X' or 'sleeping together'. The connection between the sex act and food was made visually in the movie *Tom Jones* in 1963 and, at the time, what made that scene both so comic and so provocative was that our cognitive models for having sex were not, by and large, food centred. They still aren't, although they may be in other cultures.

This criticism of Sullivan's presentation of Erickson does not mean that metaphor has no place in therapy. It certainly does. As noted already, colourful or witty metaphors may attract the client's attention and keep it, and people recall vivid language better. Extended metaphors, such as equating dinner with sex, are excellent vehicles to discuss taboo matters so that clients aren't too threatened or embarrassed in the therapy session. However, the therapist must ensure that the client understands what the metaphor is really about. In other words, at the end, a short summation should be mentioned to the effect that 'Eating dinner and making love aren't all that different.'

Ferrara[44] presents a more effective usage of therapy and metaphor. Her rationale is somewhat different from Sullivan's or other followers of Erickson. She informs us that one study found an average of three metaphors per 100 words in one hour of therapy. In order to understand the speech event in which it is embedded, this frequent usage must be understood. She feels that metaphor is an oblique, non-threatening way of talking about problems. In this, Erickson and Sullivan would probably concur.

Ferrara also points out that metaphor 'distills and compresses thoughts and feelings. It sums up global insights.' Interestingly, like Pollio et al., Ferrara found that clients often present the metaphors. The therapist can then use these metaphors to 'spin out new connections'. Metaphors, then, can be another tool of the joint production that leads to successful therapy. She also emphasizes that the mutual effort between client and therapist in creating and interpreting metaphor leads to rapport between the principals. This concurs with Lehrer's discovery in her study of meaning in wine tasting, discussed above. Creating meaning together paves the way to other collab-orative work.

Ferrara seems aware of cognitive models underlying metaphor, although she doesn't use that label. She points out, for instance, that for one client, anger is poison, fire and a weapon. She shows how a skilled therapist picks up on these models of anger and, by repeating them and asking questions of them, furthers both awareness and bonding by showing rhapsody. For instance, when Sharon, the client, says of her anger, that it is *pus* and *poison* Marian, the therapist, used a related word in her response, '...what came *squirting* out'. The image of an infected pimple or a boil is unmistakable. When Sharon describes her anger as a fire, Marian responds, '...you're afraid of finding in you ... all [that *fire*], all the anger and the *flames*'. Sharon actually overlapped here by saying 'that *fire*' at the same time as Marian, showing conversational rhapsody.

Ferrara[45] also presents a psychiatrist ratifying a patient's metaphor in a different way, by bringing it up later in the session after it had apparently been dropped. In this instance, the client, Lana, had referred to her 'crazies' early in the interview as 'an insanity tidal wave' which she can feel coming on. Although the client doesn't use that metaphor again, after several exchanges, the therapist picks it up again and expands on it, commenting that the tidal wave keeps growing bigger and bigger.[46] Such repetition of metaphor achieves the same ends as other repetitions of a client's words, and has the same effects: creating rapport, encouraging self-expression in the client, and cultivating insight.

Ferrara[47] shows individual metaphor creation by clients, such as the client who described therapy as a dance in which first the therapist takes a step, then the client, and then both are moving together. 'It's beautiful', the client concluded. Similarly, a man describing his marriage also used a metaphor for dancing, but dancing that isn't harmonious. He complained that both partners wanted to lead, so that they ended up stumbling all over each other. Again, such figurative descriptions demonstrate the degree to which metaphorizing is natural and part of every human's linguistic repertoire.

Sometimes a client's personal metaphor can cause misinterpretation.[48] One male, a salesman, had a picture of life as climbing hills. Salepeople, by virtue of their jobs, frequently experience highs and lows in their earnings. This salesman's personal metaphor for his life conflicted with two idiomatic metaphors: *over the hill* meaning 'middle-aged', and *going downhill* which is ambiguous meaning both 'to get worse', or 'it gets easier all the time' as in 'boy, he really went downhill' vs. 'then it's downhill all the way'. When coupled with *over the hill*, it is reasonable to assume that *downhill* is meant in its negative sense. At one point in therapy, the client assured the therapist that soon he would be '*over the hill* ... and it's gonna be *downhill* ... I'm just trying to hang on till that time'.

Interestingly, not only does the therapist misunderstand the client's metaphors at first, the client misunderstands the therapist's question 'When you say "*over the hill*", what do you mean?' So wrapped up is he in his own metaphor, he fails to think of the common idiomatic interpretation of that phrase. Therefore he answered in terms of his own meaning that he would soon be successful. To him, being over the hill meant that the hard times were like a hill, and once he got over the hill, he'd be doing well again. The clue, which the therapist apparently picked up on, that he didn't mean *downhill* as 'things are degenerating', but as 'things will get better', lies in his statement that he was trying to hold on till things were downhill.

This brings us full circle back to the earlier contention that each person learns and uses language individually. It is true of single words and syntactic rules. Here we see it true of the metaphors of the lives that people construct for themselves. I tried a small testing of the expression 'over the hill' on ten people under the age of 45 and all said it mean 'past one's prime'. In that context, they also interpreted 'downhill' as meaning 'getting worse'. In the above example the therapist, because she listened closely, was able to identify the client's idiosyncratic meaning to what is otherwise an idiom. She says 'So *the hill's* not bad. It's good', and the client concurs with 'Yeah', overlapping this with the therapist's 'but good'. Ferrara says that the two never resolved this misunderstanding. From the data she presented, however, the therapist's comprehension that *over the hill* is not being used idiomatically shows that the therapist is aware of the mismatch and is beginning to understand.

If a client is very threatened by something which requires talking about, tropes are a good way to discuss the subject without actively naming it, like the patient who gave an image of his marriage being a dance. The therapist can build on this extensively, extending the metaphor without directly stating what is disturbing. He or she can ask about 'stepping on toes' while trying to 'dance' in rhythm, or may speak of waltzing or tangoing, and use words like *glide* or *tripping*. If a client doesn't bring up a metaphor the therapist may be able to think of a trope that identifies the sticky situation without naming it directly. This, too, might be extended as far as it can be. The client's responses will show if he or she understands.

In sum

This chapter showed that proverbs and traditional sayings are useful for therapy, especially with addicts who need to be strongly bonded with others in their therapeutic community. Metaphors were also shown to be useful in therapy. It was also shown that metaphors are not wildly ungoverned new usages of words, but are either, like proverbs, culturally specific words with certain non-literal meanings, or are based upon culturally specific sets of concepts. As will be shown in the next chapter, the deviant speech of schizophrenics cannot be explained away as metaphor because it is not constructed, as metaphor is, on cognitive models or on metaphorical extension traceable to the actual words uttered.

Notes

1. Whaley BB (1993) When 'try, try again' turns to 'you're beating a dead horse': the rhetorical characteristics of proverbs and their potential for influencing therapeutic change. Metaphor and Symbolic Activity 8: 127.
2. Honeck RP (1997) A Proverb in Mind: The Cognitive Science of Proverbial Wit and Wisdom. Mahwah, New Jersey: Lawrence Erlbaum Associates, 124.
3. Whaley, Try, try again, 130.
4. Note that *get the ball rolling* is not a proverb. It is an idiom.
5. Honeck, A Proverb in Mind, 137.
6. Whaley, Try, try again, 133–4.
7. Ibid., 131.
8. He does not give the syllogism of which this proverb is supposedly a part, and my imagination fails me on this point.
9. Bassin A (1984) Proverbs, slogans and folk sayings in the therapeutic community: a neglected therapeutic tool. Journal of Psychoactive Drugs 16: 52.
10. Rogers TB (1989) The use of slogans, colloquialisms, and proverbs in the treatment of substance addiction: a psychological application of proverbs. Proverbium 6: 103.
11. Ibid., 105.
12. Ibid., 103.

13. I must confess that I don't know the difference between a maxim and a proverb in Bassin's usage. He doesn't define them in any way, and the examples he gives are not distinguishable. A maxim is another word for a proverb. Colloquialisms are regional usages and may or may not have anything to do with proverbs, although different regions may have their own proverbs.

14. Beck B (1987) Metaphors, cognition, and artificial intelligence. In Haskell RE (ed) Cognition and Symbolic Structures: The Psychology of Metaphoric Transformation. Norwood, New Jersey: Ablex, 9.

15. Sullivan C (1986) The therapeutic functions of metaphor. Journal of Communication Therapy 4: 138–46.

16. Szasz TS (1973) The Age of Madness: The History of Involuntary Mental Hospitalization Presented in Selected Texts. Garden City, New York: Doubleday, Anchor.

17. Beck, Metaphors, cognition, 10–11.

18. Chaika E (1982) A unified explanation for the diverse structural deviations reported for adult schizophrenics with disrupted speech. Journal of Communication Disorders 15: 167–89.

19. Forrest D (1976) Nonsense and sense in schizophrenic language. Schizophrenia Bulletin 2: 286–98.

20. Maher B (1968) The shattered language of schizophrenia. Psychiatry Today, November.

21. Hallowell EM, Smith HF (1983) Communication through poetry in the therapy of a schizophrenic patient. Journal of the American Academy of Psychoanalysis 11: 133–58.

22. Levin SR (1977) The Semantics of Metaphor. Baltimore: Johns Hopkins University Press, 31.

23. As when we say, 'Boy, he sure ate that up', meaning that he unquestioningly accepted whatever facts were told to him.

24. Lakoff G, Johnson M (1980) Metaphors We Live By. Chicago: University of Chicago Press. 25. Lakoff G (1987) Women, Fire, and Dangerous Things: What Categories Reveal about the Mind. Chicago: University of Chicago Press, 1987).

26. Lakoff G, Turner M (1989) More Than Cool Reason: A Field Guide to Poetic Metaphor. Chicago: University of Chicago Press.

27. Lakoff, Women, Fire, 381–97.

28. Gibbs RW Jr (1987) What does it mean to say that a metaphor has been understood? In Haskell RE (ed) Cognition and Symbolic Structures: The Psychology of Metaphoric Transformation. Norwood, NJ: Ablex, 45.

29. Lehrer A (1983) The Semantics of Wine Tasting. Bloomington: Indiana University Press.

30. Miller GA (1982) Some problems in the theory of demonstrative reference. In Jarvella R, Klein W (eds) Speech, Place, and Action. New York: John Wiley, 68.

31. Sternberg R, Tourangeau R, Nigro G (1979) Metaphor, induction, and social policy: the convergence of macroscopic and microscopic views. In Ortony A (ed) Metaphor and Thought. New York: Cambridge University Press, 334–5.
32. Note that this is further proof that similes and metaphors are not the same.
33. Highly esoteric metaphors may need explanation. That is the province of the rabbi explaining the Bible, the preacher explaining the Gospels, or the professor of literature. We have a term for such specialized metaphor explication: exegesis.
34. Rumelhart D (1979) Some problems with the notion of literal meanings. In Ortony A (ed) Metaphor and Thought. New York: Cambridge University Press, 83.
35. Clark H, Lucy P (1975) Understanding what is meant from what is said: a study in conversationally conveyed requests. Journal of Verbal Learning and Verbal Behavior 14: 56–72.
36. Beck, Metaphors, cognition, 13.
37. Chafe W (1968) Idiomaticity as an anomaly in the Chomskyan paradigm. Foundations of Language 4: 109–27.
38. Pollio HR, Barlow JM, Fine HJ, Pollio MR (eds) (1977) Psychology and the Poetics of Growth: Figurative Language in Psychology, Psychotherapy, and Education. Hillsdale, NJ: Lawrence Erlbaum Publishers, 143.
39. Sullivan, Therapeutic functions.
40. Ibid., 142.
41. Ibid., 143–4.
42. Turner V (1974) Dramas, Fields, and Metaphors. Ithaca, New York: Cornell University Press, 144.
43. Unfortunately, this therapy session, as described by Sullivan, has unintentionally hilarious ramifications of a befuddled couple without a clue as to why the therapist was talking about dinner!
44. Ferrara KW (1994) Therapeutic Ways with Words. New York: Oxford University Press, 129–35.
45. Ibid., 137–8.
46. Ibid., 143.
47. Ibid., 133.
48. Ibid., 136–7.

Chapter 5
Schizophrenia and therapy

The listener is told if he has ears for it what it is like to be a schizophrenic[1]

Introduction

This chapter defines what schizophrenia is and how it is manifested in a cluster of speech deviations which, together, are pathognomic of this disease. The question of whether or not such deviations should be a requirement for a diagnosis of schizophrenia is discussed. The degree to which such speech can be interpreted is debated. The aetiology of the disease is discussed in structural terms, showing that schizophrenia is both a disorder of attention and of self-monitoring. Some courses of treatment are then discussed and evaluated.

Schizophrenia and speech

Schizophrenia is an especially baffling disease for therapists. DSM-IV, p. 285 lists as its five possible symptoms (1) delusions, (2) hallucinations, (3) disorganized speech (e.g. frequent derailment or incoherence), (4) grossly disorganized or catatonic behaviour and (5) negative symptoms, i.e. affective flattening, alogia or alvolition. Two or more of the five symptoms, if present for a month, lead to a diagnosis of schizophrenia. These symptoms comprise an inordinately wide variation in behaviours for characterizing one and the same mental illness, ranging as they do from lack of speech, activity or emotion to florid behaviours often characterized by profuse verbalization of a very particular set of speech disorders (SD), as discusssed in Chaika,[2] and, for convenience, presented again below.

Whether or not these symptoms should be lumped together as constituting one disease entity is questionable, but to consider, as DSM-IV does, that SD need not be present at any time for a diagnosis of schizophrenia, seems to me to be shaky. I suggest that those with no SD have a different illness from those who do. In other words, those with speech pathognomic of schizophrenia are suffering from a different illness from those who speak structurally normally.

Walsh (1997) comments that 'schizophrenia is increasingly regarded as a disorder of language',[3] and Crow, in many writings, has presented the view that whatever causes schizophrenia is linked to the origins of language in *homo sapiens*. Although he considers mental illness as being on a continuum from depression to schizophrenia, he also considers[4] the presence of SD and Schneider's first-rank symptoms, summarized below, as necessary concomitants for a diagnosis of schizophrenia.[5] It strikes me that these first-rank symptoms are largely language-based, as they include the subjects' hearing their thoughts being echoed, or hearing voices speaking about themselves. Subjects also experience thoughts that are not their own and which they claim are being inserted into their minds. They may also experience their thoughts being shared with others without being uttered aloud. 'Thought withdrawal,' also involves language dysfunction. Here subjects claim that their thoughts have been removed from their heads. Since thoughts, to be recognized, have to be first encoded into language, these phenonema are tantamount to subjects feeling that part of their language production has been inserted, uttered or removed. If we take these first-rank symptoms along with the specific speech peculiarities – peculiarities which, in combination, occur in schizophrenia – it seems to me that language disorders are the primary symptom in schizophrenia and the absence of language disruptions indicates another illness or another point on the continuum of mental illness. The Schneiderian first-rank symptoms are perceptual dysfunctions of one's own speech. The following are dysfunctions of production.

In speech production, the following set of behaviours are pathognomic of schizophrenia, although it must be stressed that these occur during psychotic bouts and that, at other times, the patient usually speaks structurally normally. Also, there is a cyclicity to SD so that a patient in one monologue or conversation may speak normally for a bit, start rhyming or alliterating, descend into gibberish, produce word salads, and then intersperse neologisms into otherwise normal phrases. Schizophrenic speech consists of the following characteristics:

1. Neologisms

(a)   ... you have to have a *plausity* of amendments to go through for the children's code, and it's no mental disturbance of *puterience*, it is an *amorition* law.[6]

(b)   I'm don't like the way I'm *puped* today in thought ... because of the slash of my wrist like I'm was *puped* to do. I'm be *puped* tall letter I'm write to you ...[7]

(c)   He still had *fooch* with *teykrimes* I'd be willing to betcha[8]

2. Gibberish

(a)   Ulrass, Asia, Peru, arull, pelluss, Pisa, Annuell Pelli[9]

(b)   totototototototo[10]

3. Opposite speech or wrong word for intended meaning

(a) *yes* for *no*, *always* for *never*, *I do know* for *I don't know*.[11]

(b) ... but what's to say there's nothing up in that ice age that is yet to come supposedly this summer and in this winter coming up you could see quite a *recession* of them and then they come on pretty strong.[12]

4. Glossomania

(utterance of associative chains of words not subordinated to a topic)

(a)   ... Das ist **vom** Kaiserhaus, sie haben es **vom** dem **Vor**el**tern, von** der **Vor**w**elt, von** der Ur**welt, Frank**furt-am-Main, das sind die **Frank**en, die **Frank**furter Wurschtchen, **Frank**enthal, **Frank**enstein ...[13] (Here boldfaced segments show one set of chaining and underlinings show another.)

(b)   Doctor, I have pains in my chest and hope and wonder if my box is broken and heart is beaten for my soul and salvation and heaven, Amen.[14]

(c)   (in response to being asked the colour of Munsell Disc#2, a salmon colour) A fish swims. You call it a salmon. You cook it. You put it in a can. You open the can. You look at it in this color.

5. Rhyming inappropriate to the topic or occasion of discourse

(a) (in response to being asked the colour of Munsell Disc 2) Looks like clay. Sounds like gray. Take you for a roll in the hay. Hay day. May day. Help! I just can't. Need help. May day.[15]

6. Perseveration of speech forms

(a) ... when I'm not sure if its possible about the way I think I could read people mind about people's society attitude plot and spirit so I think I could read their mind as they drive by in the car sh-*will I see Paradise will I not see Paradise should I answer should I not answer I not answer* w- their thought of how I read think I could read their mind about when they pass by in the car in the house pass by in the car in the house pass by in the car by my house I just correct for them for having me feel better about myself not answer will I should I answer should I not answer *will I see paradise will I not see paradise* ...[16]

(b) You know that you knew everything everything that I wanted. You are the one who knows. It's the mother, it's the mother, it's the mother, it's the mother, it's the mother, it's the mother, it's the mother, uhm. It's the mother of her.[17]

7. Severe disruptions in syntax

(a) After John Black has recovered in special neutral form of life the honest bring back to doctor's agents must take John Black out through making up design meaning straight neutral underworld shadow tunnel.[18]

(b) ... so that's why I'm asking you could we just get together and try to work it out all together for one big party or something *ezz it hey if it we'd all in which is in not* they've been here...[19]

(c) ... you should be able to with your thought process your mental process and your brain wave you should be able to acquire the *memory* knowledge necessary as to study the bible to speak and think in a *lord* tongue you should be able to *memory* all the knowledge down on down on the page in the bible book to work for god in the mission now in the position I am in now with the *medicate* and with the hospital program. I am being helped but at the same time that I am being help with the food and *medicate* the food and *medicate* and the food and *medicate* and an the ah rest I feel that I still do not have this *I still not have* the thought pattern and the mental process and the brain wave necessary to open up a page open up the old testament and start *to memory* it the old te- the old new testament page of the bible start to have me- *memory* knowledge necessary to speak to think in the lo- speak and think in the lord's tongue.

(d) succeeded in the *pull* of a perfect crime ... framed by the artificial *insemi-nate* Detroit Michigan is in danger *of have* of World War III site Russia and Israel is *try* to drive me to approve of war against Canada.[20]

8. Disordered discourse

(In response to being asked to recall a videotaped story of a child wanting ice cream that patient had seen the previous week)   You want me to talk about – um– last week's experience I had? 'n it was funny 'is experience seems to sum up all of what's been goin' on because I've been walkin' around recitin' things. I've written to people and people been listening but then when you get down to it you've got to scrub your own dishes or else nobody's gonna and I've been so totally against the idea of people feelin' they have a ticket to carry them along because it's a ticket is not an easy trip along by no means is probably harder if you understand what I mean.[21]

Notice that several examples above display more than one kind of error. 4(a) is glossomania, but also perseveration of sounds, as shown by the underlinings and boldfaced syllables. In addition, 6(a) and (b) and 7(b) and (c) are also examples of disordered schizophrenic discourse.

Theories have abounded as to what causes such speech, although a discussion of its aetiology, which rapidly turns into a set of scholarly arguments for and against various theories, is out of the province of this book. It suffices just to point out that the speech data presented above indicate an underlying inability to organize speech structures at every level. This can be caused by at least three factors, alone or in concert. The patient is unable to focus his or her attention on the task at hand. There is a failure in the executive function of the brain which normally selects words and forms appropriate phrasing according to intent of the speaker. Finally, the patient is randomly accessing phrases which encode memories even if they don't fit the context. Perseverations also indicate problems with accessing linguistic data. It's as if the patient gets stuck for a while at certain junctures, preventing a smooth flow of articulation of ideas. I have written extensively on this elsewhere.[22]

Whatever theory one subscribes to about language production in schizophrenia, the above data show distinct structural deviations. Language is a multilevel system of meaningless sounds which are formed by rule into meaningful morphemes and words. These last are grouped together into phrases and sentences which, in turn, form discourses.

SD schizophrenics may cycle through these levels, producing errors in morpheme and word construction, yielding gibberish or neologisms. The distinction between the two is that gibberish consists of totally unintelligible strings of sounds, whereas neologisms are interspersed into comprehensible phrases and sound like words with beginnings and ends. Even if they manage to produce morphemes and words in the language, SD schizophrenics may not form them properly into phrases, or the phrases into sentences. Even if they manage these last, their discourses may go awry.

Such errors also bespeak of an inability to self-monitor speech correctly.[23] Most people make speech errors caused by faulty word retrieval or application of syntactic rules, but self-monitoring systems usually allow the speaker to self-correct them. Even in the relatively rare instances when such monitoring fails, if a hearer comments on the error, such as saying 'You mean ...', the normal speaker is able to recognize and correct it.

In order for speech to be produced, we have to posit an Executive[24] function which retrieves sounds and words, and then fashions them into phrases. We must also assume an internal monitor which prevents the executive from retrieving wrong items or guards against their being formed incorrectly. This Executive is the something that does the actual retrieval of words and phrases that encode what one intends to say. The Executive-internal monitoring system must determine the appropriateness of what is being retrieved and constructed before it is audibly expressed. Although it seems likely that an Executive below the level of consciousness is responsible for selecting the linguistic material and that an internal monitor checks it before it is uttered, at this stage in our knowledge, this is conjecture, but conjecture based upon what we know about the complexity of language production, studies of linguistic behaviours of split-brain patients[25] and research[26] into slips of the tongue. That is, we can't see either the Executive or the internal monitor, but there is no way to explain normal or abnormal speech without them.

However the final configuration of the Executive and self-monitors turns out to be, dysfunction in Executive and self-monitoring would yield the same result for schizophrenics: erroneous material constructed at every level of speech, although, usually, interspersed with normal phrasing, as with many of the examples above. However, the normal phrasing might not fit the context, as in 4(c) and 8(a). Speech is so complex that it is rare, in the absence of massive injury, for all parts of all utterances to be disordered.

The nearest analog to SD speech is that of normal people who make slips of the tongue.[27] Researchers into that phenomenon show that slips can be elicited in the laboratory by the experimenters' uttering words or showing distracting objects or pictures while subjects are talking about something else. The distracting items find their way into the subjects' speech manifesting themselves as slips of the tongue.[28] I strongly suspect that many schizophrenic deviations are caused by memories coming into focus, memories that are not pertinent to what is happening at the time of speaking and the schizophrenic is not able to suppress them, so he or she utters them. Chafe's[29] insights into how memories or present surroundings come into focus also applies here. When something does come into focus, it stimulates memories attached to the focal point of the speaker's attention, and puts them on standby status, so to speak, so they can be easily retrieved if needed.

Chafe also stressed that foci change rapidly as we talk. He was, of course, not speaking of schizophrenics. For most people, the changes themselves are still governed by the matter at hand, as a rule. If something comes into focus unbidden, the normal person recognizes this and, if it is pertinent to present or past events, may say 'Oh, that reminds me ...' or 'I've been meaning to tell you ...' At other times the information brought into focus is simply not spoken of if the speaker deems it inappropriate or unwise. In contrast, the SD schizophrenic such as the one in 5(a) above is a good example of this process gone awry. Words attached in any way to what is being said, whether they are rhyming words, synonyms, words that begin with the same sounds, memories of events, or any other possible connection come too far into focus. The SD schizophrenic then articulates them, indicating that he or she cannot inhibit what is in focal memory. This, of course, is a self-monitoring dysfunction as well as one of focus. Notice that, as Chafe's theory would predict, the inappropriate material is expressed in phrases, with one phrase evoking another, with the relationship between the phrases usually lying in the head word of each phrase. This last, the head word, is what Langacker terms the 'profiled word' (Chapter 1), the one to which the rest of the phrase adheres, such as a noun which is modified by adjectives. The noun is the head word.

Unlike Chafe's picture of short, timed bursts of speech corresponding to focal points, much SD speech is spoken rapidly without the stressed words and pausing we expect in ordinary speech, another indication of the lack of control the patient has over his or her speech. Moreover, the perseverations shown above like 'I am being help with the food and the medicate', also a prominent feature in schizophrenic speech, are reminiscent of a record getting stuck at one point. In short, there is no smooth flow of focal points here.

Self-monitoring deficits in schizophrenic speech also fit in with the Schneiderian first-rank symptoms in which patients can't tell if what they are hearing is emanating from outside or inside themselves. Long monologues like those in 6(a) and 7(c) are like speech on automatic pilot. The salient thing about such discourse is that the patient's first words start out being relevant and well-formed, but, as he or she talks, they become increasingly disordered.

What complicates this entire problem is that, when in remission, the speech of schizophrenics utilizes normal linguistic structure. It is apparently this phenomenon that, especially before the last few years, has caused some to think that the patient with disorganized speech is deliberately speaking that way. As explained above, my strongly held view is that during psychotic bouts, schizophrenics are truly SD. They have no control over their speech output. As the symptoms of the disease remit, then the patient gets more and more control over his or her speech and irrelevant associations are inhibited. As Kean[30] emphasizes, 'deviant linguistic behaviour arises as a consequence of an interaction between impaired and intact components of the language faculty'.

Crow, Done, and Sacker[31] show that one childhood precursor to adult schizophrenia is a deficit in written and oral communication, suggesting that later SD schizophrenia does or may originate in actual linguistic deficits but, since there is remittal of symptoms when patients are not actively psychotic, we still have to assume a good degree of intact linguistic ability that cannot be accessed appropriately when in a psychotic state. I say this tentatively because we badly need large-scale longitudinal studies which include long speech samples of recovered schizophrenics elicited by a task requiring them to narrate or discuss a target matter, such as describing a picture or short videoscene. Then these must be analysed by a trained linguist to see if there are deficits compared to non-schizophrenics given the same task. To my knowledge, so far no such controlled study has been done on schizophrenics who are recovered, so we sense more than know that SD subsides when psychosis remits.

In any event, no purely social theory of the origins of SD explains it. Conjectures, such as saying the schizophrenic speaks like that because he or she does not pay attention to the needs of the listener, cannot account for the peculiarities and cyclicity of this speech. Besides, any common bore fails to take into account the listener's needs, but they don't talk like schizophrenics. Indeed, non-schizophrenics usually cannot duplicate such speech even after they've heard it. The plethora of interpretations of schizophrenic speech over the decades shows how lacking in transparency the deviations are. It has taken me long hours of careful linguistic analyses to figure out what the deficits were in such speech, and how they could be characterized with precision.

Some therapists and psychoanalysts posit that schizophrenics deliberately speak as they do because they wish to be obscure or they do not want to reveal shameful secrets. If the patient chooses to utilize schizophrenic speech disorder, then we are left with the uncomfortable conclusion that schizophrenia is a wilful failure to conform to conversational rules. If this is true, it impinges directly upon therapy in two ways. If the speaker has enough control so that he or she is speaking deviantly at will, then treatment must be geared to making the patient just stop it. A very strict behavioural therapy would be in order as one would have to question if the person needed therapy or punishment for failing to conform. The problem with this is that when SD patients are presented with their faulty productions, they typically just keep on talking, or look at one blankly, or remain silent. I have never been able to get proof that a patient under-stands that he or she has just spoken deviantly, even though the patient might, at some point in the interview, apologize for stuttering. On rare occasions a patient has said that they don't speak too well, but they aren't able to say what it is that wasn't good in their speech.

At least one zealous reformer has claimed that schizophrenics are insti-tutionalized because their metaphors are unnacceptable to their psych-iatrists.[32] As we have seen, however, schizophrenic bizarre speech is not structured with the well-formed cognitive models underlying normal metaphor. My presumption is, then, that such speech is non-volitional.

The reader may recall that two of Grice's maxims for discourse are that speakers tell the truth and that they speak only of what is relevant. Neither of these, of course, is true, but hearers usually assume that they are, and that is how they interpret what is said. Thus, it is not surprising that many brilliant scholars have assumed that there is true meaning in what the SD patient has said.

For instance, the famous sociologist Goffman[33] did observe psychotics in institutions. Although I find most of his work wonderfully insightful, I find his pronouncements about psychotics not valid. No scholar, especially one like Goffman who turned his mind to so many facets of behaviour, can be correct all the time. Moreover, he was writing long before the burst in research activity in schizophrenia research of the last quarter century. Yet his writings about the mentally ill are still read in sociology and social work classes,[34] and therefore deserve comment. Goffman's apparent, but probably unconscious, adherence to Grice's maxims led him to believe that psychosis was voluntary. For instance, Goffman includes psychotic illusions under the category of **fabrications**. Fabrications, of course, are deceptions and suggest wilful intent on the part of the one who creates them. Not surprisingly, then, Goffman includes here *psychotic fabrications* (his terminology) in which the individual **deludes himself** (emphasis mine) about the nature of the world.[35] In other words, Goffman is saying that psychotic delusions must be blameworthy because the patient creates them for himself or herself. Goffman goes on to say that psychotic fabrications are atypical discourse practices that, once adopted (another word indicating agency) 'generate a continuous array of insane behavior'.[36] He actually says about those who have illusions that they actively work against their own capacity for framing discourses. Goffman offers no explanations of why anyone would want to make themselves crazy deliberately, which is what he is suggesting.

I am sceptical about Goffman's assumptions for several reasons. Years of studying speech-disordered schizophrenics, including talking to them personally, confirms my belief, as noted above, that the patient actually has no control over the kinds of speech deviations cited above. Moreover, there are analogs to the SD deviations identified above in languages and cultures all over the globe. Timothy Crow[37] claims that language disorders of schizophrenia have been found in Australian Aborigines, African Bantus, the central Borneans, the Alaskan Inuit and the Nigerian Yoruba. It is unlikely that disparate persons from such highly different cultures, speaking very different languages, could deliberately fashion this panoply of deviations[38] just because they feel like it. Moreover, this kind of speech co-occurs with other deviant behaviours, including hallucinations and delusions, neither of which are necessarily pleasant. In fact, they can be downright terrifying. What we're dealing with here is illness.

I also find it hard to accept the belief that schizophrenic speech disorder is volitional because laypersons, even those who have heard a speech disordered schizophrenic, find it difficult to impossible to repeat the structural abnormalities in schizophrenic speech. They just know that the speech is strange. Note that we are not talking about semantic peculiarities. Anyone can mimic those, but they can't generate the deviations in word and phrase structure, glossomania, and perseverations. Non-schizophrenics, especially those who never heard them, would never even think of these even if they wanted to sound 'crazy'. In my classes, when students are presented with these data, they are consistently surprised as they had never even imagined language being used this way. Even therapists who recognize psychotic speech when they hear it cannot describe what is wrong with the speech.[39] Most therapists, even the authors of *DSMIII* and *IV*, resort to vague terminology when describing schizophrenic speech, using words like *derailment* and *tangentiality* to describe it. As familiar as I have become with SD speech, I can tell others about it only from samples that I have memorized. I cannot produce original SD speech that would convince anyone who has dealt extensively with it. This may be a deficit in my own abilities but, truthfully, even when therapists discuss it, when giving examples, they too usually resort to excerpts of what they've heard. If SD schizophrenic speech is not something easily achievable by those who are most familiar with it, how, then, can ordinary people not surrounded by it produce it volitionally when they want to act psychotic enough to be institutionalized?

Then again, such speech leads one to be institutionalized. Unless one is an investigative reporter, perhaps, or a sociologist who wishes to experience how personnel treat one if they think one is insane, it is hard to believe that many people would want to be admitted to a mental institution.

This brings me to the other reason I am sceptical of the idea that schizophrenics speak crazily because they want to. There is no payback for a patient who talks this way. The wards I've visited and done studies on are humane, but hardly country clubs. Moreover, evidence suggests that patients on wards often have hostile relations with each other.[40,41] Schizophrenic deviant speech itself leads to hospitalization and, often, alienation from family and friends. It can even lead to loss of one's job, not because employers are punitive, but because the actively psychotic person can't work with any consistency and is prone to disvalued behaviours. Since their social perceptions are so faulty,[42] schizophrenics are also very difficult to deal with. Their behaviour is highly unpredictable and volatile. They are out of control, not only in speech. There are, in essence, severe societal repercussions from being perceived as psychotic and this perception is often based upon speech.

Another reason that I believe disordered speech is not wilfully produced is that recovered speech disordered schizophrenics report themselves as not being able to say what they intended while they were ill.[43] Moreover, schizophrenia is not a condition one wills oneself into gladly. The movie image of the happy deluded psychotic does not square with the agony of the schizophrenics I have met while doing research. Ribeiro[44] quotes R.D. Laing[45] as calling a psychotic bout 'a visit to the inner world', not a breakdown. This is not the place to rebut Laing or even Ribeiro's belief in him, except to note that, for the reasons cited above, I reject such views. Schizophrenics are ill. Their hallucinations can be frightening. Hearing unbidden voices in their heads, as they often do, can be terrifying. The position taken here is that the schizophrenic cannot help speaking deviantly if the illness has affected their ability to fashion sounds, morphemes, words, sentences, and discourses into coherent structures that say what the speaker wants to convey, any more than they can prevent hallucinations from visiting them.

If a schizophrenic does speak deviantly and cannot help it, then to what degree can he or she partake in therapy? Can we assign meaning to highly disorganized speech, which is another way of asking: can we hold the speaker responsible for what he or she has said while in the throes of a psychotic bout? Then, too, how can we be sure that the patient understands what another is saying? I've had patients ask me if I just said something when I've been silent. They aren't sure whether it was I or the voice in their head who was talking. It does happen that a patient seems not to understand stretches of what is said to him or her, as shown in the Dona Jurema interview below. Usually they do evince understanding of at least part of what is said to them, but whether or not they understand, their responses may not be coherent, much less cogent. The problem for therapy is 'What part are they understanding?' and 'How do they understand it?' Since actively psychotic schizophrenics seem unable to answer questions about what they've just said or about what the therapist has said, it is difficult to determine their level of comprehension. However, we must remember that speech disruptions occur mostly during the early acute phase of a psychotic episode.

I have done a study of newly admitted schizophrenics which involved their having to tell me what they had just seen on a video and then, a week later, recall what they had seen.[46] Most understood the question and gave me some sort of synopsis of what they saw. The video was very short, 124 seconds. Actively psychotic patients aren't likely to have attention spans much longer than that. Even in these short narratives, the schizophrenics showed typical SD speech deviations including intrusions of inappropriate materials.[47] The therapeutic session is certainly longer than two minutes, and the speakers aren't as constrained in a therapeutic interview as they are in narrating the short video. The less constraint on their output, the more off the track their speech is likely to become. As already noted, typically, schizophrenic speech becomes more and more deviant the longer the patient is talking. In short, there is no reliable way to measure if the patient understands the therapeutic situation, nor can one always be sure what their deviant speech means, as we shall see in the Dona Jurema case study discussed below. Some of it may be interpretable, in part or whole, and some may not. This interview, however, took place when the patient was newly admitted and in an acute stage. Two weeks later, upon release, Dona Jurema's speech was within the bounds of normalcy. We must remember when we speak of therapy for schizophrenics that we don't have to confine it to the early stages. As the patient becomes less psychotic, interventions can be, and have been, designed for prevention of relapse, for better handling of emotions, and better social interactions.

Dona Jurema

This brings us back to the questions of how much we can understand from such speech, and, concomitantly, whether therapy is possible for such disordered speakers? Actually, the first question is primary. If we can't make sense of what someone is saying or why, then therapy is not possible. Fortunately, humans have built into them the ability to understand imperfect speech, which is why we can understand small children, speakers of dialects different from our own, and foreign speakers. We can also understand people with various speech pathologies provided they are not too pronounced, as in aphasias. Can we understand everything a severely SD speaker says? Certainly, there is much we can. For instance, in 8 above, although the speaker did not stick to the topic by telling me what he had seen on the video the previous week, and although he did not use usual metaphors for certain propositions, I could still understand that he was complaining about people, probably those on welfare, who feel they have a right to a 'free ride' in life. 'I've been so totally against the idea of people feelin' they have a ticket to carry them along.' The reference to 'a ticket to carry them along' is similar to the common idiom 'to have a free ride' in life. This was probably suggested to him because the video was about a child who wanted her parents to give her money for ice cream, which her father did. The patient even gives his objection to welfare:

'because it's a ticket is not an easy trip along by no means is probably harder if you understand what I mean.' I did understand what he meant. Being on welfare may give one a free ride, but living on welfare makes for a hard life. The patient also used novel expressions to give the idea that one has to do things for oneself, 'you've got to scrub your own dishes or else nobody's gonna'. I can understand him because, although he didn't use the usual phrasing to express such thoughts, he did use phrases that could be construed the same way and he juxtaposed the imagery of 'scrubbing ones own dishes' to 'the free ride'. Tangentially, then, the patient's narration made sense.

Notice there was no gibberish and no word salad. Actually, even if there were, if enough of the verbiage is decodable phrasing, some meaning can still be derived. I shall never know what 'fooch with teykrimes' were supposed to be, but that the patient in 1(c) was talking about her pets was evident by what preceded it: mention of her cat named GI Joe and 'a goldfish, too, like a clown/Happy Hallowe'en Down'. The connection to Hallowe'en was apparently because of the mention of *clown* because *down* rhymes with *clown*. As I have shown in great detail elsewhere, words related by semantic association or phonetic similarity are often chained in SD schizophrenia in the acute stage of illness.[48] Notice that my interpretations in both of these cases stay very close to the language actually used and relates it to equivalent expressions or to well-known features of psychotic speech such as associational chaining and rhyming for the sake of rhyme. If we are going to give an interpretation of SD speech we have to account in a principled fashion for our interpretation and we must also admit that there are some portions that can't be interpreted at all, either because they are part of dense word salads consisting of words that don't seem to go together semantically, or because neologisms or gibberish aren't interpretable from the context. Patients in this state are not able to define terms when asked about them. Ribeiro[49] tries to prove that, by using frame analysis, one can make sense of incoherent speech. Frames are the schema we have for things in our culture.[50] Frames may be the physical context of utterance, like being in church or at a football game. An interview may be a frame, so is a discussion between a professor and student, or a consultation with a physician. The very fact that one is in a frame constrains what is said, how it is said (degrees of politeness), who gets to manage the topics, and what topics are permissible to raise. Goffman[51] speaks of *frame space*, the options open to a speaker in a given frame. The same words uttered in different frames take on new meaning, so that the frame in which we perceive another to be colours our interpretation of what he or she is saying.

Ribeiro analyses two interviews with a schizophrenic woman, Dona Jurema. The first was within two days of her admittance, and the second took place upon discharge 19 days later when her schizophrenic symptoms had subsided. We are here interested only in the first interview as, on the day of discharge, Dona Jurema's speech was normal. Ribeiro[52] recognizes Dona Jurema's incoherence in the first interview, and admits that 'In the opening interview the patient's contributions, for the most part, don't make sense.' Yet, Ribeiro feels, if we chunk that interview into frames, some coherence will be created. This interview is a collection of stretches of gibberish, singing, chanting, and idiosyncratic topic shifts.[53] It is true that some of Dona Jurema's speech is comprehensible, but in my estimation, it is far from coherent. Snatches of even the most incoherent schizophrenic speech typically make sense, but may still be incoherent in the entire. There is a difference between incoherence and understandable phrases. One can occur without the other. For instance, Dona Jurema repeats sentences like 'I won't allow it' and 'I've already said it',[54] but there is no mention of what she won't allow and she never references what she's already said. The latter is actually chanted three times. There are also large stretches of gibberish in her intake interview, like 'totototototo' and 'popopodedededdd'. Ribeiro[55] thinks that Dona Jurema performs different roles in this interview, acting as a child talking to her mother, sister and grandmother. At other times, she speaks as if she is her mother or grandmother. She seldom takes on the patient's role and addresses the doctor. Still, Ribeiro claims that: '*These frames carry communicative intent. In each of them, Dona Jurema remains coherent* [italics mine].' From the data Ribeiro presents, it is more accurate to say that Dona Jurema manages to utter comprehensible speech for very short segments, usually a phrase or two at a time, then abruptly changes roles or utters gibberish. In no way do these several role-playings add up to a narrative. Changes in role while talking are called changes in *footing*, and these occur in normal speech as well. In normal speech, the speaker prepares the hearer for them by noting that they are about to quote someone, by using transitional phrases, or by certain changes in tone. However, Dona Jurema never prepares us for them. She never says things like 'When my grandmother told me to do X, I would say___'. In contrast, the role shifting that Ribeiro claims is evinced simply by going from one sentence to the next. Usually, each different 'role' is played for the duration of one sentencelike phrase. The researcher interprets these as changing footing, but Dona Jurema never uses the usual devices to let us know she is going to go from being her mother to being a grandchild, for instance. Nor does she stick with any role long enough for one to be sure that she is playing a role. Her speech abounds with associational changes and random triggering of memories. What Ribeiro alleges are changes in footing actually help add up to the general incoherence of Dona Jurema's speech. Here is a sample from her speech. It is a response to the interviewer's previous two requests for Jurema's full name.[56]

(a) Patient: Let me speak because I know my full name. [baby talk] Holy Mother of God.

(b)   Doctor: So tell me your full name.
(c)   Patient: No only if you have, do you have? Oh, mama.
(d)   Doctor: Have what?
(e)   Patient: Mama
(f)   Doctor: Mmm?
(g)   Patient   Mama! Mamma! She says she has, mama. She says we can leave, mama. [here patient picks up slipper]
(h)   Then ask to be excused my child. [here patient puts on slipper]
(i)   It's like this we ask [here patient bends down and forward]
(j)   So much curiosity
(k)   They wanted to have, didn't they child ['hhh] to know about you, right child, just because ['hhh] they saw you barefooted out of doors, right child ['hhh] they thought you had

This was followed by a long burst of gibberish. Notice also that the object of *have*[57] is never supplied, although the doctor asks 'Have what?' This is no normal ellipsis because the object can't be discerned from the context. Clearly memories have been activated and inappropriately brought into the discourse. The patient never does tell the doctor her name, although her 'Let me speak because I know my full name' shows she has processed the question. Of course, her way of acknowledging it is strange. The very fact that she was asked a question means that the psychiatrist is letting her speak. Although Ribeiro doesn't mention it, (g) to (k) above seems as if the patient is hallucinating or answering to voices in her head.

Ribeiro claims that the patient does recognize the doctor and acts out a patient's schema, using language to complain, to request that she be allowed to leave, and to request attention. It is true that Dona says 'hi!' to the doctor after the doctor has called her name nine times. This is a rather belated recognition. Also, she doesn't really ask the doctor if she can leave. She tells the absent mother that the doctor says 'we can leave' (without referencing who *we* are); then, in Ribeiro's view, in the apparent guise of her mother talking to her Dona Jurema says 'Then ask to be excused my child.' Now, as it happens, Dona Jurema is herself a mother. Why didn't Ribeiro presume that Dona Jurema was talking to her absent son? It is not evident, from what she says, to whom she is talking or to whom she is responding.

Note also that these statements are out of chronological order, in that first Dona Jurema says 'we can leave' and then, in a mother's voice, says 'then ask to be excused'. Usually one asks to be excused first, and then the way is prepared for 'we can leave'.[58] Actually, the patient doesn't directly ask if she can go, although when she says 'it's like this we ask' one imagines that she is going to ask in a particular way, but she never asks at all, despite her apparently preparing us. Similarly, the phrase 'so much curiosity' is not embedded into other phrases, including the immediately previous one. It has occurred to me that 'so much curiosity' could be a reference to the fact that the doctor was repeatedly asking Dona Jurema for her name, although it could also be a reference to the mysterious 'they' who wanted to know about her because she was barefooted. The fact that she was picking up slippers when she mentioned both the curiosity and being barefooted makes me think that an old memory of being barefoot was activated by the sight of the slippers, but, of course there's no way to know. It must be stressed that Ribeiro's presentation of the raw data is exceptionally fine and complete, giving details of body motions, pausing, intonation that are rarely found in such studies. Even so, much of what this patient says is uninterpretable in any principled way.

In the putative frame of being a mother, if it can realistically be called that, perhaps the 'mother', as a voice in Dona Jurema's head, has given her daughter advice on how to ask to be excused. If 'so much curiosity' is a comment on the doctor's wanting the patient's name, it is in the wrong place in the discourse. It is not adjacent to the doctor's query. Rather, it comes after the syntactically incorrect and semantically opaque queries about 'Do you have...' This verb requires an object syntactically and semantically. I have heard only SD schizophrenics, aphasics, and some people with senile dementia make such fundamental errors in simple and common syntactic constructions. A similar one, saying *the* and then not supplying a noun to go with it also occurs in these populations, but, so far, I've never heard them in normal slips of the tongue. Dona Jurema never does answer the doctor's questions. She does talk after the doctor asks a question, but she either uses gibberish or prays or makes cryptic remarks. There is nothing here showing that Dona Jurema realized what frame she was supposed to be speaking in. Chunking this first interview into a succession of frames does not reveal coherence, as the content of each frame is so deviant. Moreover, the patient does not seem wholly aware of what is actually going on in the interview situation. As noted above, more than likely she is hallucinating and hears voices in her head. In fact, Ribeiro notes at one point that Dona Jurema is looking to the far left corner if the room, as if someone was there[59] when she calls out her sister's name.

Hallucinations and internal voices can interfere both with the patient's speaking and understanding, even with their perceptions of where they, the patients, are and for what purpose. They cannot control their speech processes well enough to take the hearer in consideration. It's not even clear how much such patients even understand what is said and what is expected of them. Their internal overload precludes intelligent participation; however, once this is quelled, as with Dona Jurema's exit interview, the patient is able to participate in a dialogue. The controlled speech Ribeiro provides at the discharge interview makes it likely that the patient could then partake in therapy. The answer to the question of whether or not we can understand an actively SD schizophrenic depends upon how much speech distortion there is. We have to go on a case by case basis. The patient in 8(a) had already been in the hospital for eight days. At his admission interview, his speech might have been far less interpretable. Patients present very different degrees of disorganization upon admittance. Dona Jurema's was profound.

A postscript to Dona Jurema's illness is that she was going to live with her sister, whom she referred to early in the interview as 'the Pope'. In this light, it is pertinent to note that Leff and Vaughn[60] found that schizophrenics have poorer recovery prospects when they go to live with family than when they go into less personal settings. They also cannot tolerate criticism at all, so, if Leff and Vaughn are correct, Dona Jurema's going to live with a sister whom she regards as the Pope doesn't augur well for recovery.

Understanding in schizophrenia

We can compare Dona Jurema with the rest of my interview with the patient in 8. After that sequence, I asked:

Do you recall the video? I took you in the other room ...

8(a) One was about I think a little girl or boy having a ball and having to be real careful about crossin' the street an' I might be mistaken I was just thinking of movies I've watched. An... -how many did we see, two or one? Just one? Yeah that was it an' it seems like what children do in their actions just exemplify what grown-ups are like an' it just gives grown-ups a better idea to think that they are necessarily better than children y'know an' I think its time to really talk now approaching 1980s and people kids goin' to college and things like that I haven't even finished ya know it's ridiculous. [laugh]

Interviewer: You don't remember the particular videotaped story?

8(b) I just remember a little girl having a ball now. That's correct – and oh okay and then the car came by or the ball was in the road and the car came by and you were supposed to think that the driver would smash over the ball am I incorrect? And then he it turns out that the little girl I don't know what her name was got the ball back and the man returned it 'n it's just like a book I read about um a really famous composer Scott Joplin I read a book about him and it seems no matter where he went people jus' wouldn't understand him um until he was dead an' then his music became popular which maybe says that people are behind the times as far as that goes. Hell, I was I've gone through a lot of bullshit this last six months. I've been kicked out of one apartment 'n you know an' moved all my stuff in and gonna leave another in jes' sound like a little baby here. We're talkin' about little babies.

Notice that the patient responds to the interviewer's prompts and responds to them in a fashion. The expression 'having a ball' idiomatically means 'having fun' in American English, and the little girl in the video is having fun getting ice cream. She is also shown crossing a parking lot to get to the ice cream parlour. What the patient did in 8 (a), is use the idiom for 'fun', but gave it the literal meaning of possessing a real ball, and then related that to the common occurrence of a ball rolling into the street.

The reference to the car coming by in 8(b) refers directly to a scene in the video in which a car indeed did come by in a parking lot. Other than that, there is no reference to or extrapolation from the video-story. There is no indication of hallucinations or inner voices either. His speech structures on the phrase and even sentence levels seem intact, although he supplies the literal meaning for the more appropriate idiomatic one, and this leads him to talk about a real ball. On the discourse level, he is not able to keep to a topic, even switching in the middle of a sentence, as when he remarks the girl got her ball back, 'the man returned it 'n it's just like a book I read about um a really famous composer Scott Joplin ...' There is no relationship between the little girl and Scott Joplin. The leap from Scott Joplin's being misunderstood and the patient's own problems with his apartment, might be an idiosyncratic connection to the patient's being misunderstood, thus being forced to leave his apartment. He ends up with the cryptic 'We're talking about little babies.' Notice that, like those who utter glossolalia, this patient went from one unrelated topic to another: the girl with a ball, to adult/child relationships, back to the girl with a ball, to Scott Joplin, to the patient's problems with his apartment, to little babies.

Had it not been an experimental procedure, a therapist could probably keep this patient on track by judicious interpolations designed to get him back to the subject at hand. Although he is clearly schizophrenic, he is not beyond talking to at this point. He understands speech and addresses all his remarks to the interviewer, not to inner voices or hallucinations, as Dona Jurema does. He is also very co-operative and responds to what is asked of him to the best of his ability. He doesn't do a good job of remembering last week's video, but that doesn't preclude his ability to converse in a controlled situation with a therapist willing to yank him back on to the topic when he starts digressing.

In the United Kingdom, speech therapists do mental health therapy, although in the United States clinically trained social workers do it. Of course, in both countries psychiatrists, psychologists, and psychoanalysts also undertake therapy. Muir[61] points out that the speech therapists are trained 'to listen and to decode and reconstruct deteriorated language...' She cites studies which show that speech and language therapists, because of their training in linguistics, have been shown to be superior in reconstructing schizophrenic speech than are psychiatric nurses. These studies apparently didn't compare psychiatrists or psychoanalysts with the speech therapists, but my own experience has been that there is no substitute for being able to listen closely to the structure of language in order to come up with a rational and principled interpretation of it. Most of the interpretations I have read or heard deal with global semantic meaning, much not derivable from the actual words and syntax used by the patient. As more and more psychiatrists are becoming aware of the importance of linguistic training in evaluating speech, this will, one hopes, assuredly change.

Therapy with schizophrenics

Despite the difficulty, various therapies can be done with schizophrenics, most of them structured and practically oriented towards attentional, social, and emotional management. Such therapies are no cure for schizophrenia. Rather they attempt to train the schizophrenic to cope with daily living and interactions with others. Those therapies reported in the literature typically focus on patients who have begun responding to their medication and who have calmed down. That is, those in the state in which Dona Jurema was at her first interview seem not be candidates for therapy at that point. When the patient is exhibiting florid symptoms as she was, uttering long stretches of gibberish, unable to pay attention long enough to attend to simple questions and being generally out of control, therapy cannot be effected, so far as I know. Certainly, two weeks later, upon her exit interview, Dona Jurema showed the attentional and verbal skills necessary for therapy.

In the following discussions of therapies aimed at alleviating schizophrenic dysfunctioning, one should bear in mind that although a therapy has a different name or a different set of expressions describing it, that doesn't make the therapies radically different or mutually exclusive. For instance, Laurie Macdonald[62] calls her therapeutic method 'an experiential constructivist therapy', terminology which Leff and Vaughn do not use when describing their emotional management techniques. However, it seems to me that they, too, could call their methodology 'an experiential constructivist therapy', and Macdonald could call hers, in part at least, 'emotional management'. Niki Muir similarly could make claim to both terminologies, as can Carmel Hayes with her Personal Construct Psychology. Each of the therapies described below is a valid possibility in training schizophrenics to reduce the effects of emotional and sensory overload and make it more possible for them to remain in control.

The attentional dysfunction shown above in 8(a)–(b) clearly has to be addressed. It has long been known that schizophrenics cannot deal well with emotional stress or emotionally laden relationships. For instance, as I noted above, Leff and Vaughn[63] show that schizophrenics who return to their families after hospitalization do worse than those who move to more impersonal environments. Hodel et al.[64] claim that 'if background stimuli are complex or stressful, people with schizophrenia worsen in their ability to appraise affect [in other people's facial expressions]'. It is likely that deficits in other abilities also correlate with stress in this population. Consequently, those actively involved in therapy with schizophrenics speak of attentional and emotional management techniques.

Niki Muir (personal communication), a speech and language therapist, explained to me some techniques she uses with schizophrenics in order to improve their attentional skills. She works with schizophrenics 'regardless of their mental state at the time', but affirms that acutely psychotic patients have to have shorter engagements and less verbosity on the part of the therapist. The treatment has to be more behavioural and less cognitive. She reports that she uses short utterances, marked facial expressions and a clear voice of appropriate volume. By the latter, I presume she means a fairly loud strong voice. I myself have noted that this is beneficial, working with even acutely psychotic patients. Once, while I was talking with such a patient, a very tall and stocky woman, she suddenly stood up and began declaiming in an extremely loud and threatening voice. To my surprise, a petite nurse walked over and said authoritatively, 'Sit down!' and the patient did, then continued talking with me. After that, I myself used firm, direct orders to help patients stay on the track of my experimental procedure. It seems to do little good to give patients in such a state explanations for why they should or shouldn't act in a certain way. They can't process them when actively psychotic, but they can respond to short, clear directives. Mrs Muir often deals with out-of-control behaviour also by withdrawing engagement to the point of looking away until they are quiet. She combines this with direct requests.

Niki Muir also introduces socially neutral topics with her patients, using topics that can be clarified and supported in a structured manner. By 'socially neutral', I presume she means that she avoids potentially emotional issues like politics, race, or the more inflammatory aspects of the news. Again, this is essential with psychotics because of their difficulties in handling emotion. Mrs Muir has a larger toolkit to work with. For instance, to help them make eye contact, she works directly with materials like objects and pictures of relevance to the individual, moving the item to the level of the therapist's face to draw the eye there. If the patient is speech disordered, and she can still understand what they've just said, she recaps or makes a précis of what has been said, but does so in clear, normal language. She does this so that the last thing the patient hears 'is the therapist's clarity rather than their [the patient's] confusion'. It appears to me that another benefit of this technique is that it is a way of telling the patient that you do understand him or her and that you sympathize. Their words are important to you.

She also uses direct self-monitoring techniques for patients who can tolerate them, such as audio- and videotaping and simple self-rating scales. Taping, both audio and video, can be potent tools in getting patients to see inappropriate behaviour. This can't be done as a rule in the earliest days of the psychotic bout. Once, I observed a patient watch a videotape of himself taken a few days before when he had been highly speech disordered and delusionary. He recognized himself on the tape, and then remarked, 'That's how I talk? No wonder nobody understands me.' I don't know if this encounter produced a cure or not, but, at the time, it certainly elucidated for him how deviant his speech was. He said that he had heard himself on tape before, but he thought the tape was distorted. (He made no comment on the delusion he was talking about on the tape: that chipmunks were bringing him secrets in a strange language. This was effected by seeds which they carried to him.)

In the study that I was doing in that hospital (Butler Hospital, Brown University's teaching facility), I was tape-recording participants and allowing them to listen to their recordings immediately afterwards. The intensity of their attention towards what they knew to be their own voices was remarkable. Some did comment on the errors they perceived in their speech but, again, in the absence of controlled studies, I can't say that such a technique would effect improved self-monitoring. This is an avenue well worth more investigation, however. To my knowledge, there have been no studies showing the long-term effects of having schizophrenics or other psychotic patients see themselves as others do. What is interesting is, in the few patients I observed, that they monitored their linguistic struc- tures in much the same terms as normals would. They did note speech errors and they did not comment adversely on stretches of speech that were well structured in terms of sentence-level syntax. However, they did not comment on hallucinatory material or verbal digressions. By saying that they did note speech errors, I do not mean to imply that they could pinpoint exactly what went wrong or even where it did. They seemed to have a global feeling that a given stretch of speech was, in the words of the patient mentioned above, distorted.

Successful therapies with schizophrenics are all based upon highly structured techniques designed to help patients keep their behaviours in check. This is not surprising, given that the speech data clearly show that SD becomes more pronounced as the situation becomes less constrained.

Brenner, Merlo and Foster[65] conducted a pilot study using emotional management therapy (EMT) on young adult patients. Preliminary results were promising. Those who underwent EMT showed fewer relapses and better social integration than the control group. In EMT, 'people learn how to cope with realistic situations through repeated practice in everyday situations'. Young patients also showed improvement in cognitive functioning. Because groups can be so stressful for schizophrenics, Brenner et al. started with individual therapy and then added one or two people more per group. Individuals were taught relaxation techniques. These were as simple as whistling a tune or looking in a shop window. Besides discussing their physical and cognitive reactions to stress, fear, and excitement, patients engaged in role-playing in which they coped with such situations. Whenever possible, Brenner and his colleagues allowed subjects to suggest the topics used in therapy. The discussions and role- playing also helped patients to improve 'significantly in terms of ability to differentiate affective stimuli and in reduction of psychopathological symptoms'. It seems to me that this works so well because routinizing everyday social situations and drilling patients in what to say and do gives them behaviours to fall back upon without becoming stressed out. By having the patients suggest the topics, they are assured of being given solutions relevant to their own lives. Like Niki Muir's attentional exercises, this is a very flexible and practical approach.

Two other therapies, both aimed at changing specific behaviours, also deserve consideration. The first is Personal Construct Therapy. Carmel Hayes[66] specifically disavows that Personal Construct Theory, hereafter PCP, is more than the acquisition of behavioural skills. She claims that it is a theory of personality, namely that the personality is developed through a series of constructs. PCP recognizes that when people experience something, they create a construct, by construal, which they then apply to new situations, so that their behaviour is guided by their constructs of the world. Although this is undoubtedly true in most instances, it seems to me hard to say that this is true of an actively psychotic person. The whole point with them is that their constructs have apparently collapsed. They are far too disorganized to be construing outward events, even when they are capable of distinguishing between outward and inward events which, often, they are not. Of course, inner constructs are not obvious and cannot be worked upon except by what is evinced in outward behaviour. Advocates of PCP recognize this, and after denying that the approach is behavioural, Hayes says 'PCP is, therefore, an attractive approach when working with clients with mental health problems because of its focus on what people do rather than on what they are...'[67] Indeed, the goals she states are, in essence, behavioural ones, such as 'control: ability to initiate action and respond to others and to determine to whom we speak and what we say'.[68] Hayes claims that interpersonal difficulties stem directly from 'a person's particular construction of their social world. It assumes that these constructions are the best available means of anticipating events and that they, and the consequent "social skill deficit" represent the client's way of life.'[69]

On this view, then, the therapist's job is to encourage the client to explore alternative constructions of their lives, rather than simply trying to train them in specific social skills. As already noted, this approach is certainly valid for some mentally ill people, such as depressives, and perhaps even for schizophrenics who are in remission, but it does not seem a viable method for patients exhibiting florid symptoms of acute psychosis. It would seem to be best after therapies designed to improve attention and to manage emotion have been employed and their hallucinations and delusions have subsided. This is not to disregard PCP as a therapeutic technique. Its emphasis on teaching patients not to elaborate on roles such as being 'schizophrenic', 'depressive' or a 'poor communicator', but rather focusing on other, more successful, areas of their personalities, is very important. So is PCP's emphasis on group therapy focusing on basic communication skills, teaching members to express emotions, opinions and ideas, and giving feedback to others. Thus members of the group learn to see things from each others' point of view and to clarify their views of themselves.[70] Again, however, schizophrenics have to be stabilized first before PCP can be employed.

It might also be noted that PCP implies that schizophrenics have made themselves schizophrenic by the way they have chosen to construct experience. The problem seems quite different. Experience has been restructured for them by the illness itself. Tim Crow[71] has shown that this disease strikes in every culture and in every kind of culture, evincing the same set of symptoms, which include an inability to focus outside of the self while in the acute phase. Hayes concludes that 'If we are to help someone make communicative change, then the more we understand of the way in which his or her world is construed, the more likely we are to be able to suit the therapy we offer to individual needs ...'[72] This is true of a wide range of mental problems, such as depression, but the psychotic must first learn to manage his or her emotions and be able to attend to the matter at hand. For schizophrenics, behavioural techniques like Niki Muir's and Brenner et al.'s seem to be the first lines of approach, along with medication, of course. Then PCP group therapy, and the similar Neurolinguistic programming, discussed below, can be employed.

Laurie Macdonald[73] also suggests highly structured techniques to effect behavioural changes in schizophrenics. She calls her methodology 'Neurolinguistic Programming' (NLP). Like PCP, described above, NLP also seeks to understand the process by which an individual experiences his or her world, but it more specifically targets the communication diffi- culties of schizophrenics. NLP offers a structured framework within which the patient can function, recognizing that the patient does not have a high level of communicative competence, especially while in a psychotic state. Whereas PCP speaks of the leader of group therapy as a 'facilitator', NLP clearly speaks of the role of the therapist, and expects this to be active. Like PCP, NLP recognizes that the patient's model of the world may be quite different from the therapist's, but recognizes that this is due to dis-orders of 'perception, interpretation and under- standing of social understanding'.[74] The term *programming* is descrip- tive of this methodology. It consists of very direct questions calling for short answers. The therapist's job is to take the patient's responses as the basis for the next question. By so doing, NLP allows the therapist to help patients become motivated to certain ends and to make perspective shifts in cognition.[75] Macdonald is well aware of the importance of achieving rapport with the patient, and elaborates on what she terms 'pacing' and 'leading' to this end. Pacing involves the therapist's use of the same or similar language patterns as the patient uses. This leads the patient to 'experience a sensation of being "understood"'.[76] Certainly, this does not mean that the therapist should suddenly start speaking gibberish or rhyming inappropriately, or use any of the deviations of schizophrenic speech noted above. Rather, the therapist asks questions or makes comments which utilize the comprehensible portions of the patient's statements. She gives examples like

Patient: I need help.
Therapist: *What* do you need help with?
Patient: I'm being forced into it.
Therapist: *Who* is forcing you into *what*? [italics indicate emphatic stress]

She also shows how rephrasing can clarify issues. For instance, she notes that nominalizing, turning verbs into nouns, 'has the effect of turning an active process into a static non-changing or changeable event',[77] so the therapist can rephrase such nominalizations into active verbs, which leads to a conceptualization of a viable, changeable process. This insight is very much in line with Langacker's cognitive grammars described in Chapter 1. For instance,

Patient: He did it because of an argument.
Therapist: Something occurred as you were *arguing* that caused him to do it.

Space, and the copyright rules, don't permit a full explication of the linguistic techniques that Macdonald illustrates, but all, such as those above, take their cue from what the patient has said, and all are aimed at specifying agents and processes, such as asking '*Who* did it?', '*How* do you know what he meant?' or '*What kind of love* doesn't she have?' (in response to 'She doesn't love you'). The value of such an approach is that the language probing itself is quite concrete, forces the speaker to be precise and, by choice of syntax, helps patients see that change is possible.

Macdonald does recognize that with schizophrenics, this technique is a complement to other treatments, but is a great aid to 'the construction or reconstruction of a person's ability to perceive and respond to social situations'.[78] She sees it as a brief form of focused psychotherapy, but I would add that it is clearly also a re-education in speaking clearly, specifying agents and causes, and re-examining personal constructs, such as 'Nobody loves me' or the like. Certainly, the more the therapist listens closely to the patient's or client's actual words, using them in response, and the more the therapist keeps the therapeutic situation structured, leaving as little room as possible for digressing, the more efficacious treatment will be, especially for schizophrenics.

There are also purely psychoanalytic treatments of schizophrenia which depend upon classic Freudian notions of Oedipal complexes, repressed homosexuality, transference, countertransference, and the like, but these, like all classic psychoanalysis, involve years and years of therapy, years a schizophrenic doesn't have and frequently doesn't have the money for. Moreover, there is no proof that this kind of analysis cures psychoses (or even neuroses). That is, psychoanalytic techniques have not been subjected to studies with control groups with judges blind to the treatment each group received. Such judges would have to determine if the analysed group showed greater improvement in terms of lessening of psychotic episodes and of improvement in social attitudes and behaviour. The problem is that, given the length of time traditional psychoanalysis takes, such studies are simply not feasible. In contrast, the methodologies described above are shorter termed, and can be subjected to comparative analysis with other methodologies or even by treatment with medication alone, as we saw with Brenner et al.'s validation of EMT. That is, the interventional behavioural therapies discussed here can be demonstrated to show patient improvement or lack of it. Moreover, the therapist can expect to see if a treatment like PCP, EMT, or NLP is working or not relatively early on, and can switch to another therapeutic technique. This is not to say that psychoanalysis doesn't work for at least some patients. It is just that it can't be proven to work, and has the practical deficit of requiring years of treatment.

In sum

This chapter first laid out precisely what is meant by schizophrenia and precisely what deviations comprise specifically schizophrenic speech. Since schizophrenia is partially a disorder of attention, it was argued that therapy for schizophrenics must be structured. Unlike traditional psychoanalysis, which stresses that the therapist intervenes minimally in the patient's speech output, the methodologies described here require the therapist to intervene to keep the patient on the subject at hand, at the same time helping to bring him or her to new realizations and new personal constructs of the world.

It was also shown that before psychotherapy can be brought into the treatment of schizophrenics, the worst of the psychotic bout has to be quelled, usually with medication, but once the patient is stabilized enough to work with a therapist, techniques of emotional management and speaking practices can be introduced. Except for techniques specifically geared to teach the patient attentional strategies, the therapies for schizophrenics are also efficacious for clients and patients with other disorders. Depressed patients and clients, for instance, can also benefit by being asked to name specific agents and causes. They, too, can be brought to examine self-defeating statements like 'Everyone is against me' or 'I never have good luck.'

Notes

1. Forrest D (1976) Nonsense and sense in schizophrenic language. Schizophrenia Bulletin 2: 289.
2. Chaika E (1982) A unified explanation for the diverse structural deviations reported for adult schizophrenics with disrupted speech. Journal of Communication Disorders 15: 167–89; Chaika E (1974) A linguist looks at 'schizophrenic' language. Brain and Language 1: 257–76.

3. Walsh I (1997) Conversational skills and schizophrenia: an exploration. In France J, Muir N (eds) Communication and the Mentally Ill Patient. London: Jessica Kingsley, 99.
4. Crow TJ (1998) Nuclear symptoms as a window on the relationship between thought and speech. British Journal of Psychiatry 173: 303–9.
5. Ibid.
6. Vetter H (1968) Language Behavior in Schizophrenia. Springfield, Ill: Charles C Thomas, 189.
7. Herbert R, Waltensperger K (1980) Schizophrasia: a case study of a paranoid schizophrenic's language. Applied Psycholinguistics 1: 85.
8. Chaika E (1974) A linguist looks at 'schizophrenic' language. Brain and Language 1: 257–76.
9. Brown J (1977) Mind, Brain, and Consciousness. New York: Academic Press, 43.
10. Ribeiro BT (1994) Coherence in Psychotic Discourse. New York: Oxford University Press, 7.
11. Laffal J (1965) Pathological and Normal Language. New York: Atherton Press, 31–5.
12. Rochester S, Martin J (1979) Crazy Talk: A Study of the Discourse of Schizophrenic Speakers, New York: Plenum Press, 247.
13. Maher B (1972) The language of schizophrenia: a review and an interpretation. British Journal of Psychiatry 120: 9.
14. Forrest, Nonsense and sense, 289.
15. Cohen B (1978) Referent communication disturbances in schizophrenia. In Schwartz S (ed) Language and Cognition in Schizophrenia. Hilldale, N.J.: Lawrence Erlbaum Publishers, 29.
16. Notice that 7(b) shows the same perseveration. This particular monologue went on at greater length, with the underlined portions being repeated at intervals.
17. Ribeiro, Coherence in Psychotic Discourse, 276.
18. Lorenz M (1961) Problems posed by schizophrenic language. Archives of General Psychiatry 4: 603.
19. Chaika E (1990) Understanding Psychotic Speech: Beyond Freud and Chomsky. Springfield, Illinois: Charles C Thomas, 221–2.
20. Herbert RK, Waltensperger KZ (1982) Linguistics, psychology, and psychopathology: the case of schizophrenic language. In Obler L, Menne L (eds) Exceptional Language and Linguistics. New York: Academic Press, 85.
21. Chaika, Understanding Psychotic Speech, 221–2.
22. Chaika E (1982) A unified explanation for the diverse structural deviations reported for adult schizophrenics with disrupted speech. Journal of Communication Disorders 15: 167–89.
23. Chaika, Understanding Psychotic Speech, 30, 58; Frith C (1997) Language and communication in schizophrenia. In Communication and the Mentally Ill Patient. London: Jessica Kingsley, 13–14.

24. Chaika E (1995) On analysing schizophrenic speech: what model should we use? In Sims A (ed) Speech and Language Disorders in Psychiatry. London: Gaskell, 55; Morice R (1995) Language impairments and executive dysfunction in schizophrenia. In Sims A (ed) Speech and Language Disorders in Psychiatry. London: Gaskell, 62–6.

25. Gazzaniga M (1992) Nature's Mind: The Biological Roots of Thinking, Emotions, Sexuality, Language, and Intelligence. New York: Basic Books.

26. Baars BJ (ed) (1992) Experimental Slips and Human Error: Exploring the Architecture of Volition. New York: Plenum Press.

27. Ibid.

28. Dell G, Reich P (1977) To err is (no longer necessarily) human. Interfaces 6: 9–12.

29. Chafe W (1994) Discourse, Consciousness, and Time. Chicago: University of Chicago Press; Chafe W (1998) Language and the flow of thought. In Tomasello M (ed) The New Psychology of Language. Mahwah, New Jersey: Lawrence Erlbaum Associates, 93–111.

30. Kean ML (1980) Grammatical representations and the description of language processing. In Caplan D (ed) Biological Studies of Mental Processes. Cambridge, Mass: MIT Press, 242.

31. Crow T, Done J, Sacker A (1995) Childhood precursors of psychosis as clues to its evolutionary origins. European Archives of Psychiatry and Clinical Neuroscience 245: 61–9.

32. Szasz TS (1973) The Age of Madness: The History of Involuntary Mental Hospitalization. Presented in Selected Texts. Garden City, New York: Doubleday, Anchor.

33. Goffman E (1974) Frame Analysis: An Essay on the Organization of Experience. Cambridge, Mass: Harvard University Press, 84.

34. In America, social workers with the degree in Master of Social Work frequently do psychotherapy, and are often exposed to Goffman's work on the mentally ill and mental institutions.

35. Goffman, Frame Analysis, 112.

36. Ibid., 246.

37. Crow, Nuclear symptoms, 304.

38. Chaika, A unified explanation; Chaika, Understanding Psychotic Speech, 3–27.

39. Lorenz, Problems posed by schizophrenic language, 603–10

40. Abrahamson D (1997) Social networks and their development in the community. In France J, Muir N (eds) Communication and the Mentally Ill Patient: Developmental and Linguistic Approaches to Schizophrenia. London: Jessica Kingsley, 153–4.

41. Goffman E (1968) Asylums: Essays on the Social Situations of Mental Patients and Other Inmates. London: Penguin Books.

42. Hodel B, Brenner M, Merlo G, Teuber F (1998) Emotional management therapy in early psychosis. British Journal of Psychiatry 173: 128.

43. Chapman J (1966) The early symptoms of schizophrenia. British Journal of Psychiatry 112: 225–51. Also, in conversations with three schizophrenics while they were in remission, I was told spontaneously by them that they could not say what was 'in their heads' or what they intended, and often couldn't make sense of what was said to them. Two of these conversations occurred after I had given talks at scholarly meetings and these persons came up to speak to me privately afterwards.

44. Ribeiro BT (1994) Coherence in Psychotic Discourse. New York: Oxford University Press, 238.

45. Laing RD (1967) The Politics of Experience and The Bird of Paradise. Harmondsworth, Middlesex: Penguin, 110.

46. Chaika E, Alexander P (1986) The ice cream stories: a study in normal and psychotic narrations. Discourse Processes 9: 305–28; Chaika, Understanding Psychotic Speech, 17,131,134,183–90.

47. Chaika, Understanding Psychotic Speech, 190.

48. Chaika, A linguist looks at 'schizophrenic' language, 257–76.

49. Ribeiro, Coherence in Psychotic Discourse, 25–35.

50. Brown G, Yule G (1983) Discourse Analysis. New York: Cambridge University Press, 238.

51. Goffman E (1981) Forms of Talk. Philadelphia: University of Pennsylvania Press, 230.

52. Ribeiro, Coherence in Psychotic Discourse, 57.

53. Ibid., 58.

54. Ibid., 8.

55. Ibid., 192.

56. It must be stressed here that I do not even attempt to reproduce Ribeiro's superb and detailed notations showing pauses, changes in voice quality, and the like.

57. In English and most European languages, it is obligatory to put an object or verb form after *have*. This is as obligatory as putting a noun after *the*. In the data I've collected, only severely speech disordered psychotic patients have omitted such things as the object of *have*, and I have also heard it from an aphasic patient and those suffering from senile dementia, but never from a manic, even in pressured speech, nor in a slip of the tongue by a non-impaired person. This doesn't mean that these people never make such errors. I just haven't been able to find any examples of it.

58. Temporal misorderings in schizophrenic speech are quite usual. For instance, in The Ice Cream Stories study of narration, one patient told me 'She ate the ice cream and took it home.'

59. Ribeiro, Coherence in Psychotic Discourse, 7.

60. Leff J, Vaughn C (1985) Expressed Emotion in Families: Its Significance for Mental Illness. New York: The Guilford Press.

61. Muir N (1997) Semantic pragmatic disorder and the role of the speech and language therapist in psychiatry. In France J, Muir N (eds)

Communication and the Mentally Ill Patient: Developmental and Linguistic Approaches to Schizophrenia. London: Jessica Kingsley, 118.

62. Macdonald L (1997) Neuro Linguistic Programming as an experiential constructivist therapy for semantic pragmatic disorder. In France J, Muir N (eds) Communication and the Mentally Ill Patient: Developmental and Linguistic Approaches to Schizophrenia. London: Jessica Kingsley, 139–52.

63. Leff and Vaughn, Expressed Emotion in Families.

64. Hodel B, Brenner M, Merlo G, Teuber F (1998) Emotional management therapy in early psychosis. British Journal of Psychiatry 173: 128.

65. Ibid., 129, 132.

66. Hayes C (1997) Applying personal construct psychology. In France J, Muir N (eds) Communication and the Mentally Ill Patient: Developmental and Linguistic Approaches to Schizophrenia. London: Jessica Kingsley, 127–38.

67. Ibid., 131.

68. Ibid., 127.

69. Ibid., 131.

70. Ibid., 136.

71. Crow TJ (1998) Nuclear symptoms as a window on the relationship between thought and speech. British Journal of Psychiatry 173: 303–9.

72. Hayes, Applying personal construct psychology, 137–8.

73. Macdonald, Neuro Linguistic Programming, 139–52.

74. Ibid., 139–40.

75. Ibid., 141–2.

76. Ibid., 143.

77. Ibid., 145.

78. Ibid., 151.

Chapter 6
Telling a life

People create and maintain social, cognitive and emotional order in their lives by their narrative construction [creating self].[1]

All human beings are guided by the stories they construct.[2]

Introduction

This chapter shows how people make sense of their lives by creating personal narratives. These narratives, told and retold, can reinforce the individual's irrational fears which cause agoraphobia or paranoia, but they can also be used to manipulate others in the family. Sociolinguistic studies of how people use language to project a persona and to save face are discussed. Here we listen to the stories told by an agoraphobic, a paranoid recluse, a perpetual prisoner, an unemployable epileptic and barflies.

Everybody has a story

Everybody constructs their personal reality by the narrative they shape for themselves about their lives. As Bamberg[3] says, they tell their lives. When new events occur, they fit them into their existing life story according to the persona they have created for themselves. Continuity of self is maintained and created by constructing a narrative of one's life.[4] Language is the greatest human resource for representing and structuring events in our lives, as well as for letting others know who we are, or who we want to be. Personal life stories may be used to show others that one is worthy even though one doesn't live up to society's expectations. Lamentably, some of these stories that people construct may seriously impair their ability to function as members of a family or to function in society at all.[5] It is unfortunately true that some life stories form a negative framework into which all subsequent events are fitted, thus fulfilling the dysfunctional personal narrative.

Sometimes people are able to readjust their life stories in order to accommodate new events. In so doing, they reinterpret old ones. One such instigator of reinterpretation, but not the only one, can be psychotherapy. Such therapy can be seen as a way of re-authoring one's life, co-authoring it with a therapist.[6] Mrs Jenny France, a speech therapist[7] for many years at Broadmoor Hospital in the UK, feels that therapy is teaching people new linguistic resources so that they can not only gain self-esteem, but change their responses to others. Additionally, Pollio et al.[8] claim that what the client learns in psychotherapy is a style of communication and a strategy for problem-solving. In short, therapy is a way of learning that one is a worthy member of society and how to cope with society.

Obviously, people have varied reasons for entering into therapy. Some do so because they need help in maintaining or creating better social relationships with other individuals, either at home or at work. Others enter therapy because they feel as if they are not functioning optimally in society. They may feel humiliated by their failure to succeed by society's norms. Some, of course, come to therapy because they are court-ordered to do so. In any event, they may have deep feelings of inadequacy and shame, feelings that are difficult to acknowledge, much less to express to others.

All humans have ego needs. They must feel that they are worthwhile individuals in order to function constructively in society and to be at all at peace with themselves and with other people. If therapy is seen as a re-authoring of one's life, then one component of that re-authoring has to be concerned with helping the client or patient understand that he or she can be a capable, respectable member of society, even if he or she does not hold a prestigious job position. Another portion of the reauthoring must be concerned with teaching the client or patient how to deal with others in a non-confrontational or non-submissive manner. This sounds almost boringly evident, but too often we all forget how easily bruised egos can be and usually are.

Those who can't find a place in society often feel deep shame. Such people go to great lengths in their stories to preserve their self-image as models of what society says they should be. A person can be virtually crippled by what they perceive as society's rejection. Few manage to escape unscathed by social rejection and, often, their only weapon against it is the stories they tell. What it all boils down to is that people have strong ego needs and, one way or another, language is utilized to help achieve them. Charlotte Linde,[9] in her study of life stories, comments:

> we use ... [our self-constructed life] stories to claim or negotiate group membership and to demonstrate that we are in fact worthy members of those groups, understanding and properly following their moral standards.

Before examining narratives themselves, it is important to consider the accents and dialects that people use because these, like the narratives, are based upon ego needs as well as on social realities. I spoke of dialects in Chapter 3 in terms of the therapeutic situation. Here we shall see an example of a dialect used to project a persona. The dialect a client uses is not always going to be important in the therapeutic setting, but it can be. If a client uses an ordinary working-class dialect or an educated dialect, it may just mean that he or she is an ordinary working-class person or an educated one. It's when the accent doesn't fit the social situation of the speaker or it is hypercorrect that we sense it is telling us something.

Ego and social behaviours: some socio-linguistic background

The stories people tell about their lives are stories mirrored in other facets of their speech practices, as in the dialects they adopt, or the speech routines they initiate. For instance, Clive, presented below, spoke with an accent that belied his true station in life, and Meg, also presented below, used phrases of subservient begging as a way of commanding her husband. For both of these people and for very different reasons, such behaviours fulfilled ego needs. We shall be examining more closely the stories people tell to create themselves as worthy members of society.

Using language for ego-boosting is seen in all people who are down and out, or whose egos have suffered serious damage by their not being able to achieve respect in their families or society. For those who can't live up to societal expectations, ego-satisfaction is often done through narrative, such as the tall tale, or an exaggerated telling of one's life. I make it my business to listen to street people asking for handouts. I don't listen just to the request, but to the stories, given half a chance, many of them blurt out as they beg. One, for instance, as I was fishing for coins, rapidly assured me he almost had a chance at a contract in pro basketball. Others assure me that they had jobs but other people poisoned the boss's mind against them. These tales are told hurriedly in barely audible voices, the voices of shame. Erving Goffman[10] claimed that the more a person is not acceptable by society's central values, the more often he or she feels compelled to tell his or her sad tale. That is just another way of saying how important 'face'[11] is to everyone.

That face needs are fundamental human needs is shown by those who are institutionally outcast, as African Americans often still are and Jews once were. Typically, such groups develop entire structures within which they can achieve ego-satisfaction. Those groups in society who are denied access to prestige positions often develop speech routines and activities in which their members have a chance to be ranked highly. The traditional competitive oral performances and constant verbal gaming of African American males comprise one manifestation of this.[12] In addition, the churches of African American culture have always been another outlet for displaying morality and concomitant verbal prowess for those who felt, justifiably, that they were demeaned by the dominant society. Both the street performances of Black youth and the church have provided prestige and enhanced ego satisfaction for those who could not get it in the society around them. A man could be a janitor, called 'boy' by the white folks he worked for but, on Sundays, he was an influential man, called Deacon, an honourable title. Although rejected by the dominant society, African Americans could still be validated as worthwhile individuals within their own groups by being accomplished speakers and devout church members. This is not to say that males chose both roles. Often, they chose one or another.[13] Another path to success was to become a preacher. It is no accident that so many of our most prominent African-American leaders, like Martin Luther King, Jr., were preachers. That was one of the few prestigious positions open to African Americans. Before the Civil Rights Movement, very few could become physicians, scientists or professors because so few universities would accept Black students.

Over the centuries the Jews of Europe, despised by the mainstream society and confined to ghettoes or restricted rural areas in eastern Europe, gained their ego satisfaction by refining their scholarly skills in religious studies. Prestige was achieved and maintained by how well they understood Hebrew, how much of the Bible and its commentaries they knew and how well they could argue their positions. The overt insults and violence Jews were subject to was counteracted by the respect they could gain within their communities by their religious scholarship and piety. In addition, the Jews of eastern Europe maintained their own language, Yiddish. This was used at home and in ordinary conversation and reinforced bonding and solidarity within the group.[14]

As these groups have gained fuller and fuller access to participation in society, including access to prestige positions, their speech behaviours have conformed more and more to those of the already dominant groups. Yiddish is no longer spoken by most Jews, who have become assimilated into the general culture. The scholarly skills of the ghettoes of Vilna or Warsaw have been exchanged for skill in science and other secular studies. Educated middle-class African Americans are often quite unaware of the verbal gaming of their predecessors like **toasting** and **playing the dozens**.[15] They, too, often modify the African American dialects which are used for social bonding and speak like mainstream middle class Americans. However, since large numbers of African-Americans are still not as assimilated to the dominant society as Jews, for instance are, they still retain to a greater degree distinctly black speech activities and music, such as **rap** songs (which actually are the descendants of the earlier black oral productions known as **toasting**[16]).

Since **face needs**, that is, ego-satisfaction, help determine what stories we tell about ourselves, not surprisingly face needs are built into everyday speaking routines, such as greeting, requesting, complimenting and questioning. The pragmatics of daily interaction in every society we know of is established in such a way so that within groups members' egos will not be unduly damaged. We don't usually command directly, for instance, because a direct command entails that the one being commanded is inferior to the commander. Consequently, we pragmatically effect commands by asking polite pseudo-questions like, 'Excuse me, but would you please....'[17] Face needs are prime determiners in how we frame invitations, criticisms, compliments – in short, all of our social interactions.

If a speaker doesn't show regard for another's face needs, then an insult or rude remark has been given. It is true that under the guise of 'kidding' people can insult each other, but even here, there are bounds on the topics of such kidding, which William Labov[18] termed 'ritual insults' (see also Chaika[19]).

Greetings, which the anthropologist Malinowski[20] called **phatic communication**, are a way of reassuring members of society that they are worthy of recognition and still a part of their social group. The address forms in greeting, depending on the given society, either exaggerate the speaker's respect for the person addressed by using formal titles, or emphasize the strong social bonds between those in the interaction such as by using mutual first names. In languages which still preserve the distinction between formal and intimate 'you' forms, choosing one form over the other helps determine social intimacy or distance. Either way, face needs are met.

Although narrative is the focus here, other facets of language use are also affected by the need for individuals to signal identity. Understanding this can be of great value to a therapist. Too often, professionals presume that if a person speaks with a non-standard dialect, that person is simply stupid or coarse. Rather, that person is showing in his or her speech his or her allegiance to a given group or is presenting a certain persona identified with that group, such as being macho. Intelligence has nothing to do with it. All dialects of all languages are equally complex. The alert therapist can tell much about clients just by listening to the forms of speech they use, even when the speakers are trying to use standard forms. As we shall see, they can't do so consistently, although the attempt shows they are trying to conform to the therapist's world.

Investigations of entire communities have proven to us how important speech is in signalling identity. For instance, in all modern communities there are variable ways of pronouncing words. Typically, just a few sounds within the local language or dialect differ from group to group. There are many reasons for variable pronunciation. First, as Leslie Milroy[21] showed, in Northern Ireland people who see each other frequently and have strong social ties signal this by their pronunciation and word usage. In fact, the single most predictive measure of dense social networks is similarity in speech patterns.

Earlier, Labov[22] showed that in any community there is more than one way to pronounce certain words. He called these **speech variables** and correlated each with specific social groups. Actually, what Labov found is that people are not wholly consistent in their pronunciations. That is, the variables which demarcated groups were not an absolute set of pronunciations, but the percentage of time individuals used one pronunciation or another. He demonstrated that New York City speakers showed their feelings of social identity by the variable ways they pronounced the vowels in words like *man, gas, coffee* and *talk*, as well as by the way they pronounce the initial consonant in words like *throw* and *though*. Another variable was whether or not they pronounced the /r/ before consonants in words like *park*, or the final /r/ in words like *car*. The final /r/ would be pronounced by some speakers only if the next word began with a vowel, but if it was the last word in a sentence or the next word began with a consonant, the /r/ was not pronounced. These rules for /r/ dropping are virtually identical with those for southern British speech.

At the time he was studying New York speech, the social structure of the city was changing rapidly. As this was changing, so was New York City speech. The speech changes correlated consistently with the changes in social stratification. For instance, whereas older New Yorkers pronounced words differently according to ethnic ties, such as being Italian, Jewish or Irish, younger speakers did not use those ethnic markers in their speech. Rather, their pronunciation divided along lines of education and race. Ethnicity was no longer the prime determinant of social grouping. Education and race were. For example, educated speakers pronounced /r/'s a greater percentage of time than did the uneducated. Educated pronunciations were recognized as prestige forms by almost all members of the community that Labov tested, whether they used them often or not.

Later, after collecting the original data, Labov played people tapes and asked them to indicate when they heard the pronunciation they used. What he found was that people who used a prestige pronunciation no more than 30 per cent of the time claimed that they used it all the time. In other words, people monitor themselves as speaking prestigiously when, in fact, they actually speak like those they identify with. If the latter cohort doesn't consistently use prestige forms, neither will the person tested.

Labov et al.[23] found that even hardened gang members in Harlem reported themselves as using prestige forms that they don't. For instance, Labov et al. devised what they called the Vernacular Correction Test for these gang members. Robbins, the African-American field worker, read sentences to the group and had them, as a whole, discuss whether or not they used the forms presented, forms which we know from many other studies to be features of what is now called Ebonics (Black English). One of these is the possessive marker which is often omitted in Ebonics. Therefore, one sentence read to the boys was 'That's Nick boy.' Boot, one of the roughest, toughest members of the gang, immediately shouted out three corrections, all with the possessive intact,

That's Mr. Nick's son
That's Nick's son right there.
Do you know that's Nick's son.

Later, however, when asked directly about whether or not he used another feature of Ebonics, Boot responded

Some people that don't speak correc' English do. Calvin little brother do.

Note that (a) Boot is concerned with presenting himself as speaking correct English and (b) despite his earlier protestations, he omitted the possessive on Calvin. Being seen as one who conforms to social standards is important for just about everyone's ego, even those who seem most removed from the standards of the middle class.[24]

Labov's findings have been replicated many times. In the video *American Tongues*, an excellent sampling of American dialects, several people, all speaking with very different accents, claim they don't have an accent and speak neutrally, like newscasters. Americans typically believe that having no regional accent is desirable, and, for some odd reason, they think that paid newscasters are the reference point for how one should speak.[25] The findings of pragmatics in general and of dialect studies are pertinent to our understanding of human behaviour including that in therapeutic situations. This is because people adopt an accent or other features of a dialect as a way of projecting a certain persona. A young male in the United States who wishes to be seen as tough and sexually aggressive typically adopts working-class or Black English features of speech. If, instead, he wishes to be seen as educated, as belonging (or wishing to belong) to the professional class, he will, in contrast, utilize the words and pronunciation associated with lawyers, physicians, teachers and the like.[26] Many people command more than one dialect, using each in different circumstances to elicit different reactions from others.

This quick summation of how people choose to speak has its counterpart in the stories people tell about themselves. The correlation between a person's accent in a therapeutic interview and the stories that person tells in the interview is well illustrated in an encounter with a man I here call Clive.

Clive

While collecting data at Broadmoor Hospital in Berkshire, UK, one subject, Clive, walked into the room, carrying a large, impressive novel. Mrs Jenny France, the speech therapist who mentored me, and I were both duly impressed, as no doubt we were intended to be. In all of my experience in eliciting speech data from the mentally ill, I had never had a patient bring such a tome to the taping room. We commented favourably on his choice of reading material. He beamed, and told us he loved reading, especially the masters, like Shakespeare and Dickens. He also consistently spoke with a distinct educated southern British accent, with one revealing exception. He consistently failed to pronounce the sounds spelled as *th* in words like *both* and *mother*, substituting /f/ and /v/, respectively. The importance of this apparently innocuous fact will be seen shortly.

Clive proceeded to tell us the high levels he had achieved in school, on the academic track, of course. What made this all the more impressive was that the suburb he claimed to have been raised and gone to school in was quite upper class. By his accent and his claims of exam scores, Clive was clearly presenting himself as a person of substance and education.

Later, he did happen to mention that he somehow hadn't actually taken the requisite exams, so he never actually attained the academic levels he claimed but, he assured us, he would have if he had taken the exams. When I asked why he hadn't, his answer was foggy. He more or less implied that it was an arbitrary decision on the headmaster's part but, he continued, he was going to another school anyhow. In fact, we elicited from him that he had actually gone to many schools because, he said, his mother kept moving, getting different jobs and the like. Still, if he hadn't actually taken his A levels, or lesser exams, and done superbly on them, he was presenting himself as one who could have, and this was clearly important to his ego; hence, the upper-class accent, the book he toted, and the claim that he loved the classics.

Mrs France did tell me that the suburb he named as his childhood residence was quite upper class. I did ask him if he had playmates and friends at school. 'Oh, yes,' he assured me. Not only did his formal history, presented below, belie this, but so did the mispronunciations mentioned above. Throughout most of the English speaking world, pronouncing *th* in words like *both* or *throw* as [θ], or the *th* in *mother* as [v] or *this* as [ð] is a sign of uneducated speech. Sociolinguistic studies have long verified that children learn to speak like their friends, regardless of how their parents speak. Had Clive been friendly with the children of the suburb he named and been accepted by them, he would have spoken as they did, including using the educated pronunciation of the two *th* sounds. As it happens, it appears that these sounds, if not learned in childhood, are difficult to manage with any consistency in adulthood, although other accent features are easily changed.[27] In short, these pronunciations alone contradicted Clive's claims of friendship with children of this suburb. Then, too, was the strange bit about the headmaster's purportedly not allowing Clive to take his exams.

Clive proceeded to tell us about the morning's events. In Chapter 1, we have already seen that one can encode one's experiences in such a way that one is never an agent, the one who initiated an action or process. Instead, one is always, grammatically, a patient, one to whom things just happen. Clive fits into this pattern. After presenting his story, I shall present the facts from his records about his schooling and his behaviour while hospitalized and in jail. These show the degree to which a life story can be used for ego gratification.

After establishing his love for reading and his academic credentials, Clive announced 'I'm quite upset today. I've had a very bad morning.' 'Why?' I sympathized. 'Well,' he said, 'I went to the bathroom to take my bath and it was filthy. The man who just used it didn't clean it. So I asked him to please go clean the tub so I could use it. He called me a "black bastard", so I went to the nurse and complained. Then I went to my room. When I came out later, I went back to the bathroom, and it was still dirty, so I complained again. I kept complaining, but no matter how long I waited, the bathroom wasn't cleaned, and I was getting angry.'

'Weren't you also humiliated?' I suggested. Whereupon, he musingly repeated, 'Yes, humiliated.' 'Good for me,' I thought. 'I gave him a new way to see the source of his anger, or at least one source.'

He continued, 'Finally, I went to my room. My slippers were there. There was marijuana stuffed in one of them. When I came out of my room, there were policemen lined up facing me, with DOGS! They brought dogs, attack dogs. I was humiliated.' (As he used the word *humiliated*, he glanced over to me.)

Yes, I had given him a new word with which to describe his feelings, but it didn't contribute to his view of how or why events occurred to him. He was able to incorporate it into the way he perceived how things happened to him. We chatted some more. He shed no light on the mysterious circumstances of the marijuana in his slipper or the sudden presence of a phalanx of policemen with dogs. According to his telling, these things had simply happened.

Clive then admitted that he had actually been transferred from the maximum security facility where I was doing research to an interim 'halfway house' on his way to being discharged into the community. Unfortunately, he had been returned the day before from the less secure house to this very secure facility. He gave no explanation for his being remanded to Broadmoor, and, intermittently through the conversation, expressed his desire to see a doctor, as he was convinced that once such a meeting took place, he was sure he'd be released to the community. That is, he'd be on the streets again.

In response to my direct question about his return to the present hospital, he replied that there was some kind of ruckus in his room at the halfway house while he and his roommate were there together. Nevertheless, the roommate had been released into the community but he, Clive, was sent back to this place. Upon persistent questioning, Clive implied that it was the roommate who caused the unnamed trouble and that he, Clive, had nothing to do with it.

'Why was the other person allowed to go into the community and not you?' I pushed.

'I don't know. He was just picked.'

Note that the passive form 'was picked' allows the speaker to avoid the mention of an agent, and the adverb *just* indicates 'chance'. Things just happen or just don't happen to Clive. It's all random. He's not responsible.

This was his way of assuring me that it was simply a matter of chance that someone who made trouble was allowed back into society, and Clive, who reported that he merely 'happened' to be 'in the vicinity' of where the disturbance was, just happened to be returned to this hospital rather than being released as his roommate was. Life, to hear Clive tell it, was just a series of inexplicable unrelated events in which he always got the short end of the stick. Despite his earnestness, it was clear to me that he was not at all likely to be released, even though he was polite, soft-spoken and seemingly quite reasonable – during the interview with me.

His final comment to me was that he was going to live in a mansion as soon as he was out. Even before this clearly delusional statement, I had already figured out that much of his narration was a fantasy. Part of his fantasy was that he wasn't an agent or a cause of anything that happened to him. Things just occurred for no reason. Perhaps his need to salvage his ego, to save face, caused him to deny responsibility. He had to present himself, undoubtedly even to himself, as someone to whom bad things happened for no reason whatsoever. His world was not one of cause and effect. His world was a chaotic place in which things just happen, few, if any of them, good.

It was not only the words he used to tell his implausible story that told me this. The syntax of his sentences did, as, of course, did the omissions from his narrative, like what happened before he went into his room to cause the staff to call for the police with canines. Why weren't the staff interested in helping him get the bathroom cleaned? What did he say to them – or, for that matter, to the patient who refused to clean up and called him 'a black bastard'? It certainly was more than passingly odd that he made such a fuss about a dirty tub, but never commented on his reaction to this highly insulting epithet. What did he feel when he was called that? What did he do or say to the person who uttered those words? Did he do anything to cause those words to be thrown at him?

I was already convinced by his own statements, or rather by what he didn't say, that Clive was probably violent, even dangerous, and must have caused quite a disturbance on his own that morning, not to mention that he must have been responsible for the trouble that landed him back at Broadmoor from the halfway house

After our discussion, I reviewed Clive's extensive case history. As I suspected, it revealed a life of violent and even vicious attacks on many people in many places, starting when he was about 10 years old. Clive's records show that, far from having a stellar academic career, and, far from being an innocent bystander at violent events, he had had serious behavioural problems from childhood onwards. At school, he was a bully, noted for aggressive outbursts and much truancy. His education was further disrupted by appearance before criminal courts. He had been involved with psychiatric services from an early age and was diagnosed as schizophrenic at the age of ten. Later, he had eleven appearances before Criminal Court before his first conviction at age 18.

Ironically, Clive described himself as being placid and loving. Not so surprisingly, the records say that he saw himself as a victim of injustice. They also report that when in hospitals, he constantly argued with people over changing TV channels, sitting on 'his' chairs, locking bathroom doors, and not leaving the bathroom clean. His actual behaviours did not jibe with his own personal life story. Sadly, for instance, although he claimed his mother was loving and caring, in actuality, she herself was schizophrenic and depressed and unable to care for any of her children. All were in foster care at an early age.

Once, during one of his numerous hospitalizations, he hit a staff member and then filed an official complaint against the staff member. This is reminiscent of the old joke about the boy who killed both his parents and then asked the court for clemency on the grounds that he was an orphan. The reports on Clive evaluated him as 'lacking in insight', 'doesn't have foresight', 'takes a random view of life' and 'there was a gulf between Clive's view of his problems and the view taken by his carers'.

His indignation about the bathroom, in itself, was revealing. Mrs France, the speech therapist, and the staff themselves said it was quite usual for someone to leave the bathroom somewhat untidy, so that the next occupant had to do some wiping up. There was nothing particularly gross about the tub when Clive went in, but perhaps it was a blow to his fragile ego to have to do any cleanup. It has also occurred to me that his actions can be viewed as an example of Clive's attempting to boost his ego by commanding another; that is, it could be seen as an attempt to establish himself as socially superior to the previous bather.

Clearly, adequate treatment for Clive should concentrate on his failure to see his involvement in what occurred to him. He has to be made aware of his agency, of causation, and of the consequences ensuing. His choice of sentence forms shows his view of his world, but without understanding that he himself is an agent, he can never be cured of his violence. The problem, of course, is that he has so thoroughly constructed an image of himself as a refined, intelligent, peaceable person that it is hard to see how to get him to look at his own role in what happens to him. Perhaps he has to be taught to rephrase some of his own sentences, making them active rather than passive, for instance, or to see the differences in agency in related sentences like 'The rose died' vs. 'The rose was killed.'

I do not minimize the difficulty of such an undertaking as it would involve crumbling the defensive walls he has built up over the years to make himself seem worthy in his own eyes. Whether he, or others like him, can ever allow this to happen is uncertain, for it would then mean admitting to guilt when, clearly, the self-story has as one of its aims evasion of guilt. Certainly, Clive's case shows how one shapes a self through one's words, a self that is completely at odds with one's actual world.

Nate

One needn't have such a dreary childhood as Clive apparently did in order to have low self-esteem. A former neighbour of mine, Nate, a cultured, well-educated scion of a high-achieving upper-class family, suffered from very severe epilepsy, so severe that it impeded his ability to work, a very embarrassing situation for him. In truth, he had never held a job in his life. He had managed to get one once, as an orderly in a home for the aged, but was let go on his first day of work when he had a seizure. Yet, part of being a worthwhile member of society, for him, apparently was to hold down a job, no matter how menial. Consequently, his conversation was peppered with repeated stories of how he almost got certain jobs, but bad luck always intervened. He himself never mentioned the experience at the home and avoided all mention of his epilepsy.

One oft-repeated tale was about the time that he waited all day in a reception area of the offices of a potential employer, apparently an acquaintance of his family. However, Nate was never called in for an interview. He waited to no avail. Afterwards, at some social gathering, the 'prospective employer' told Nate, 'I didn't know you were outside or I would have sent for you right away.' The allure of this story for Nate was clearly that someone was willing to hire him, but did not only because that person 'didn't know' that Nate was waiting for an interview for the job. The fact that any child could poke holes in this story is beside the point. What is the point is that Nate felt so compelled to tell this story over and over, even more than his other 'I almost got a job' stories. Clearly, this is because a family friend actually said he **would have** called him in for an interview, and, to Nate, this was tantamount to his actually being hired. At any rate, it was the closest he had ever come to a job, except for the aborted experience at the home. Telling the story of almost being hired apparently enabled him to justify himself as a worthy member of society. That is, Nate was willing to work and, except for fortune, he would have got a job. That his disability prevented him from holding a job even if he got it never was mentioned.

All in all, however, Nate was lucky. He came from a wealthy enough family so that there was a trust fund for his upkeep, and he had a loving stepmother. His father and biological mother were both deceased, but still he was not alone in the world. He had been sent to prestigious private schools as a boy, although he was not able to complete college. His desire for work did not flow from financial needs, but from his desire to be a man in our society, and in our society a man is defined by his job. In this instance, the fiction developed to protect Nate's feelings of self-worth is so benign that it would, in my eyes, be an act of cruelty to point out that if the man wanted to see him and give him a job, he would have.

The barflies

For his term paper, a student of mine, Robert Walling, visited neighbour-hood bars when those who had no jobs would be whiling their afternoons away. The bars were in stable neighbourhoods and most of the people working or patronizing them had known each other for years, sometimes their entire lives. Walling quickly found out that the barflies were delighted to have a new ear to tell their stories to. They actually deliber-ately sat down next to him just for the chance of speaking to him. He had to ask nothing. He found patterns of conversation, in his words 'designed to reinforce and stabilize egos'. The pattern was usually quite simple. First, the speaker started with a criticism of the current government, society, or sports figures. Apparently, this served as a way of establishing the man's superiority to those in power. An unfavourable comparison of the past to the present was then made. This was not surprising, since these barflies always claimed that their glories were in the past. Finally, the speaker gave a sketch of his past life and, if he had children, he might describe their achievements as well. When Walling investigated by interviewing the bartender and other patrons of the bar, he found that the life sketches were untrue, but not wholly so. There was always some germ of truth in these tales. Two snatches of these stories suffice to show how they built up egos.

Both of these stories were told in Providence, Rhode Island by natives of that area. In the following stories, The Outlet Company, now defunct, was still the largest department store in the city, and the Biltmore was the finest hotel. One man who many years ago had driven a city bus for ten months until he was fired for drunkenness claimed:

> I was a bus driver and a damn good one too. My wife used to work at The Outlet and now my two boys drive truck for them.

The bartender confirmed that his boys were doing no such thing, nor as their father also claimed, was it likely that they could have gone to college since they had not graduated high school in the academic track. Another oldster who had been a janitor at The Biltmore, an elegant hotel, claimed:

> I worked at the Biltmore. You name it and I did it. There wasn't much in that place that I couldn't do. That used to be the best hotel in southern New England. All the big shots who came to Providence stayed at the Biltmore [shows autographs from Jack Benny and Jack Dempsey]. Pretty impressive, huh? I talked to those two for about an hour apiece. Ya, they were great guys. I still remember what Demps told me, 'You got to fight to win in this world.' I'll never forget those words and that was almost forty years ago ... When I had my big job with the Biltmore I never complained once.

Note the use of a pseudo-nickname, Demps, to indicate familiarity or intimacy with the great fighter. For these men, part of the reason for going to bars seems to be to have a chance to tell their stories, to present themselves as worthwhile people.

Esther

Esther was born in Ukraine around 1906: Jewish, a girl, and obviously precocious, none of these particularly welcome attributes at that time. Worse yet, as soon as she began to walk, she did so with a pronounced limp because of a malformed hip. This was seen as a defect and as a further example of her unworthiness even by her own family. Simply being Jewish meant that she had to take verbal abuse from her Christian neighbours. Like African Americans prior to the Civil Rights movement in the United States who were often called 'nigger' to their faces, Jews in the Ukraine were called 'Zhid' and worse. They also witnessed on several occasions public murders of Jews and massacres, not during the famed pogroms, but by marauding soldiers during the Russian Revolution. Not surprisingly, she attributed the label Anti-Semite to virtually all Christians. My intimate knowledge of both her life and her stories derive from the complete tape recordings I made of her narratives over the span of about ten years, all with her knowledge.

Esther was also called a gimp and her walk was made fun of by other children even after the family migrated to America. At home, her family didn't try to hide the fact that she was potentially unmarriageable, both because of her leg and because of her biting retorts to teasing. It was deemed a great shame to have an unmarried daughter in this culture. In this they were, fortunately, wrong. Esther may have limped but she was beautiful and, when younger, could still be charming. She had no problem finding a husband.

She learned early to defend herself with her verbal quickness, which, by the time I knew her, was highly developed. Her remarks were unfailingly cynical. She was so sure that everybody she met disliked her on the spot, so that her way of saving her own face was to attack the person verbally. She literally could construe 'Hello. How are you?' as an insult or as another's attempt at finding out something bad about her. At family gatherings, she frequently took somebody's innocent remark as an insult and retaliated, often in loud, angry shouting. Finally, her cousins no longer invited her to weddings or bar mitzvahs, a situation she could never understand. This was the severest punishment anyone could deal out in the family-oriented culture she was raised in. It amounted to the practice of **shunning** by the Amish. She complained bitterly about being excluded from the family *fraylachs* (Yiddish for *parties*). 'Why me?' she would ask. 'I always give good gifts. I gave a good gift to X [the last wedding she had been to]. I've been sentenced without a trial.' She often reiterated, 'I've always been so good to everyone in the family, and look how they treat me.' She definitely did not correlate her scenes at weddings with the lack of subsequent invitations. To her, there were no scenes. Like Clive, she was never at fault. The difference was that, in her mind, other people were actively mean to her. To Clive, things just happened. Esther was just defending herself when others unfairly attacked her verbally. Eventually, Esther was almost completely alienated by her family, except for two brothers who visited her occasionally and one niece, me. Fortunately, she did have a devoted husband to care for her. By the time she was in her forties, she had ceased seeking people out, even her family, although she spoke of them incessantly. She also ceased going to movies, restaurants, or other forms of entertainment.

By the time she was in her fifties her life was highly circumscribed. Because she had been mugged while living in New York, she feared going through many neighbourhoods, even rural areas, even after moving to Rhode Island, a small New England state. She left her apartment only to go to the doctor, to Senior Citizen's Meal Sites[28] and, once a month, to venture across town to a particular delicatessen which carried the kind of herring she liked. Except for the doctor's visits, all of these events produced a good deal of angst.

The Senior Citizens Meal Sites were apparently filled by her enemies. Esther claimed that nobody wanted to eat with her and Al (her husband). They said terrible things about and to her, although she was never able or willing to say what exactly what the others had said, and all were, in Esther's words, Anti-Semites. Never did she quote one of these offensive remarks, Anti-Semitic or not. The deli trip was dangerous because she might get mugged again. Although she felt safe in her apartment, she was convinced that the manager and other residents disliked her, so she had no social contact with them at all. Had she ever gone to a psychiatrist, which she wouldn't hear of, she would have been diagnosed as both paranoid and agoraphobic. Her profile fits the DSM-IV symptoms of those diseases.

A visit to Esther was highly predictable. There was no topic of conversation per se. If one tried to talk about what one was doing or where one went, one would be met with a blank stare, followed by one of Esther's stories. Collectively, these were clearly life stories. They were so hardened in form that they never changed. Each of the stories that showed how badly Esther had been treated was repeated on every visit. Occasionally, the good stories of life in the old country could be elicited, but they would quickly be followed by the rest of her repertoire. One measure of how pathological her storytelling was can be seen by considering the more usual changes in an individual's story as discussed below in the section 'They lie'.

She repeated the same stories over and over all through the years. One set involved her life in the Ukraine. Somehow, over the years, she had forgotten the harsh realities of that life and her stories of life there were idyllic, all about going down to the village common land to herd the family cows home, the enormous size of tomatoes grown in the fertile soil, the time the young bull got in the back hall and wouldn't let the children out of the house, the sight of her grandfather saying his morning prayers while pacing back and forth across the floor. There was no mention of the massacres and vicious treatment of Jews which had forced emigration to America.

In contrast, the stories of her life in America were quite different. These had two themes. The first, not surprisingly, were about her accomplishments. These were ego-building. The second was about how everyone mistreated her despite her goodness and generosity. Both sets of stories had to be listened to on each visit. From her husband's casual remarks, it appeared that she constantly recounted them to him as well when they were alone. These multiple retellings served to circumscribe her life, reminding her again and again why she must stay aloof from various people and stay away from new experiences which could prove dangerous. The stories had such power that new ideas and experiences could not be presented to her. She not only told her life story, she lived it.

There were several stories in each set. The first story line was simple. I call it the 'I did it despite ...' story. She wanted to go to high school, but her father said, 'You don't need a high school diploma to diaper babies.' Therefore, she didn't go. However, years later, having moved to New York, she went to night school and did get her diploma, despite her father. A satellite story to this one was how she got her 'derivative citizenship papers'. She, like her older siblings and mother, had originally been listed on my grandfather's citizenship papers. Esther wanted her own papers. Everybody, especially her sister, said she couldn't get them, but she did and recounted in great detail how, against all odds, she defeated bureaucracy and spited her sister to boot.

Both of these stories were about how people always tried to foil her success, but she showed them. Sadly, she also frequently said wistfully that she wished she could play the piano, but her father wouldn't buy one because, again, he said, 'You don't need to play the piano to diaper babies.' Each time she told me this, I always said, 'Why didn't you buy or rent a piano and take lessons when you were on your own?' The response unfailingly was a blank stare, a short pause, and then her resumption of one of her other stories. I suspect that she never bought a piano because if she did, and then couldn't learn to play it well, her ego couldn't have withstood the blow. She recognized the greater complexity of playing the piano than of getting a high-school diploma which depended on reading and math skills she already had, or than getting her own citizenship papers. The irony of her father's remarks about diapering babies is that Esther was never able to have any, a source of great sorrow to her. She saw this as another defect in her body, one worse even than the limp. This, too, might have been a factor in her wanting not to be friendly with people. If she were friendly, she would eventually have to admit she could never have children, another blow to her ego.

A third tale involved her going to concerts when she was young, concerts given by a prestigious Jewish choir in New York City. Since she had a beautiful soprano, almost coloratura voice combined with great natural talent, she thought of trying out for the choir. With fear and trepidation, and after many false starts spread out over two years, she finally auditioned and made it. This story always ended with a refrain of 'Can you believe it? I made it and I can't read a note of music. Everybody is always surprised that I can't read music.' Since she was often asked to sing at the Senior Citizens' Meal Sites, she also, after recounting in detail what she sang, took up the refrain 'Can you believe it? Nobody believes it, but I can't read a note of music.' It sounded as if it was she who was so unfailingly astonished that she had any ability, or that she didn't believe that anyone would find her accomplished in any way.

Her fourth source of pride was that she was trilingual, a not uncommon occurrence in Jews from Ukraine. She spoke Yiddish, Russian and, of course, English. She demonstrated her proficiency in Russian by recounting a meeting with a Polish person at the Meal Site and asking him in Russian to pass the sugar. He was able to understand her Russian. This story, too, was prefaced with 'Can you believe it ... I haven't been there [Ukraine] for so many years and I can still speak it!' She would say, 'Everybody is always surprised that ...' of this accomplishment as well as of her singing.

A fifth ego-boosting story was of how she got her job as a cashier. Although this was relatively low-paying work, it certainly was steps up from the jewellery factory work she had done before. In order to get the job, to prove to the reluctant boss that he should hire her, she worked with no pay for a full day, never making even one mistake.

The sixth story is partially an ego-booster, but always led into the 'everybody mistreats me' set. Esther boasted, 'I can make a nickel do the work of a dime.' She also alluded to having large amounts of money in US Savings Bonds. She had been earning her own living since she was a young teenager and contributed to the family's upkeep. This was no mean accomplishment. Her father didn't work and died very young. In addition, Esther enabled her younger brothers to go to college, medical school, and graduate school despite holding the relatively low-paying job as a cashier. Of this she was justifiably proud. 'Would you believe it? I worked as a cashier by day and did home work[29] and sent them both to school!'

Although she was proud of their accomplishments, she was very bitter that, after they got their degrees, they didn't shower her with love, affection and undivided attention. Both had the nerve (her word) to get married and have families, who came first with them. According to Esther, both sisters-in-law offended her greatly. Details were never given, but one instance was alluded to repeatedly. In this, Esther went to visit her brother who was living in Newport, Rhode Island, a seaside town. When she got there, his wife said there was no place for Esther and her husband to sleep and all they were offered to eat was a can of tuna fish. This story ended with the refrain, 'I made him a doctor. I made her a doctor's wife. That good for nothing ...' The upshot was that she never visited again. Notice that nowhere did she say that she was invited to visit in the first place. The brother in question was just starting his private practice and was living with his in-laws who had a very tiny house. There was no place to stay, I'm sure. Although she visited him in her mind constantly, she never visited him in person again. Whenever his name or his family's was mentioned, out came the Newport story complete with abusive words about his wife and the refrain, 'And I made him a doctor ...'[30]

Similarly, she did not speak to her only sister for the last 40 years of her life. If Sarah's name was mentioned, Esther always immediately impugned her sister's character, alternating this with tales of what wonderful things she, Esther, had done for Sarah.

No attempt was ever made to make the above accounts cohere and they could be told in virtually any order. The maltreatment she received was always uncalled for, although the details were always sketchy. In Esther's mind, her not speaking or seeing her relatives was thus always justified to the listener. Since the listener never asked for such justification, the fact that she felt compelled to give it anyhow shows how much Esther must have felt that it was wrong to cut herself off from one's siblings. Of course, in her mind, their actions led her to abandon them. She was raised in a culture in which strong family ties were stressed.

She didn't ever see her husband's family either. Her explanation for this illustrates how she was able to turn very innocent statements into insults or direct attacks upon her person. Two years after her marriage, Esther told her in-laws that she was going to quit work. The mother-in-law asked, 'Why?'– whereupon Esther flounced out of the house and forever after refused to speak with or see her in-laws. She wouldn't even let her husband go visit his mother. Why? Esther's explanation was 'Al and I were trying for a baby. She had to know? She wanted me to keep on earning money so I could give it to her.' Actually, the mother-in-law's single word *why* in no way implied she wanted money. In fact, Esther never gave her mother-in-law money or anything else. Perhaps the mother-in-law merely wanted to know if she was finally going to be grandmother. In any event, her innocent question lost her her son. Esther wouldn't allow him to so much as call his mother on the phone.[31]

Although she does not fit the profile of a schizophrenic in DSM-IV, like schizophrenics, Esther could not bear close family relations. Leff and Vaughn[32] demonstrated that schizophrenics who go home to their families do worse than those who don't. They especially cannot tolerate criticism. Since Esther's paranoia led her to see every innocent comment as a criticism of her, then dealing with family, her own or her husband's, was clearly so painful that she had to find a way to be cut off from them.

Also, despite the fact that she felt that all Christians hated Jews,[33] for the last forty or so years of her life she managed always to live in remote enclaves in which she and her husband were the only Jews. My guess is that, had Esther lived in a 'Jewish' neighbourhood and been rejected by other Jews, she could not have borne the ego damage. Rather, she lived among Christians, who *de facto*, in her mind, automatically hated her because she was Jewish. She could bear what she perceived as their 'slings and arrows' and blame her lack of friends on the fact that they were Anti-Semites. In any event, she never had anything to do with any of her neighbours, and she was convinced that they and the apartment manager constantly said bad things about her behind her back because she was Jewish.

As noted above, she did go the Senior Citizen's Meal Site in her neighbourhood every day. There, too, she was sure, nobody wanted to sit with her, so she and Al had to sit alone. Her reasons for going were 'to get out a little'. Also there was entertainment by members of the group after the meal. Esther got up and sang old standard love songs and, of all things, Christian hymns. Although Esther felt the people didn't appreciate these, still, by her report and Al's, they always asked if she would sing. Yes, she always prefaced her narration of her singing at the sites with 'Would you believe ...' and 'They can't believe I can't read music.' It was as if, by singing to these (in her mind) hostile people, she was showing them, just as she had shown her father she could get a diploma. Also, like the barflies' exaggerations discussed above, the singing was an ego-booster.

For the last thirty years of her life, every conversation with Esther was a repetition of the same stories of abandonment, betrayal and hatred. The same scenes played and replayed in her mind. Her accomplishments like singing were presented as anomalies, things to be astonished at and she presented herself as one who helped out others, but was then rebuffed. There was never adequate explanation given for the 'insults' of others, what made them insults, and why they were always directed at her. Again, like Clive, no connection was ever made between her behaviour and the consequences of it. The same tales were told over and over, and with each retelling, her feelings about her family and other people were reinforced. She truly wrote herself a life story of misery and maltreatment, but one which still allowed her to present herself as a worthy person.

Meg

Capps and Ochs have broken new ground in the linguistic analysis of the mental disorder *agoraphobia*. DSM-IV categorizes *panic disorder* separately, as some agoraphobics do not get panic attacks. Esther, for instance, fits the definition of an agoraphobic, but she never had panic disorder. Meg, the agoraphobic whom Capps and Ochs interviewed, however, did. If she was in a place that called forth her agoraphobia, she responded with a severe panic attack. Lisa Capps and Elinor Ochs were able to interview Meg over a period of two and a half years. They tape-recorded each session, later analysing the entire sequence. The sessions consisted mainly of Meg's tales of her agoraphobia and subsequent panic attacks. Because they had the tape recordings to analyse and listen to over and over, several things became clear that wouldn't have been had they simply looked at a therapist's notes or even sat in upon therapy sessions. Meg's recorded narratives were their primary data and these narratives, like Esther's, became the causal factors in the agoraphobia, describing why and how Meg herself experienced what she did. The tapings allowed Capps and Ochs to see how Meg's use of syntax both revealed Meg's feelings, and also helped reinforce her agoraphobia, thus verifying Johnstone's[34] (Chapter 1) research into the unique way we use the syntactic resources of our language.

Meg repeats her stories of her panic attacks over and over, not only to the researchers, but to her children and family. Her stories are very vivid. She keeps each experience alive by retelling it, often in the present tense, and by using what Capps and Ochs[35] term 'a limited set of adverbs and adverbial phrases that denote the unexpected and the unaccountable', such as 'all of a sudden', 'out of the blue' and 'unaccountably'. These adverbials also show that Meg feels as if she is gripped by panic for no reason. She is a victim of a force beyond her control. When she is in one of these situations, such as riding on the freeway, she desperately begs her husband to get her out of there and uses forceful words such as *agony* to describe her 'desperate, pleading rendition of her troubling thoughts'.[36] She describes herself as feeling *helpless* and *trapped*, and *visibly shaking*.[37]

As one goes through the stories she recounts, however, certain constancies come through. In most, Meg has given in to her husband's request to go somewhere, but then, while on the road, 'out of the blue' she feels panicky and then implores her husband to get her home immediately. Capps and Ochs notes that, in each instance, she did not want to go to wherever it was, but did because he asked. They also realize that her panic attacks are highly controlling. She may feel out of control but 'When Meg produces directives such as

I've got to get out *now*. I feel *terrible* [italics theirs]
William, can we get *out* of here?
Can you please get *off* here?

she imposes her own agenda on others.'[38] That is, all that fear and panic winds up being highly controlling. Capps and Ochs think that Meg suffers from a communicative disorder, such that she can't say 'No' when first asked, but defers her 'refusal' until they have started their journey. They feel she has to learn to say 'No' when she is first asked. It seems to me, rather, that two purposes are served by Meg's consenting to go or do what her husband wants and then having a panic attack while they're doing it. One, as noted, is that Meg controls others by her agoraphobia. Two, she does so without relinquishing her status as a dutiful wife.

As Linde[39] claimed, people want to feel as if they fit society's dicta. Relations within a family are part of social expectations. In this instance, for Meg's generation at least, society dictates that a good woman is submissive to her husband. If she were to refuse his requests, then, of course, she would not be a dutiful wife. Consequently, she behaves like a dutiful wife and goes. When she has the panic attack that will control William, she uses wording like

I *begged* William, '*Don't* get on the freeway

or

... I just *can't*. *Please* humor me. *Indulge* me.

It seems clear to me that the very drama of the words she uses to control William also are words used to beg a superior, to plead with one, so that, even when controlling, she is doing so as an inferior who has to beg her superior. She remains every inch the submissive wife.

Although Capps and Ochs don't discuss this aspect of Meg's behaviour, another pattern becomes clear as one reads the entire account of Meg: the theme of being trapped by being a woman and having to fulfil a woman's role in this society. In almost every anecdote, Meg portrays herself as having to do something housewifely, when the husband's request disturbs her plans. For instance, her first freeway attack occurred when Meg was busy getting the house ready for Christmas, baking cookies, wrapping gifts – a very housewifely thing to do. Then, when William wanted to go visit some out-of-town relatives in a nearby hotel, Meg didn't want to go as she had too much to do, but she went anyway. There was a traffic jam on the freeway, and Meg, in her own words, felt trapped and had a panic attack which caused her to beg William to get off the freeway and back home.

Interestingly, one of her first panic attacks didn't involve William going anywhere. What happened was that Meg was nine months pregnant, but had cooked William a supper which he did not like. Meg became furious at William's spurning the meal. She wanted to leave the house, so angry did she become, but felt she couldn't because she was nine months pregnant. Her disproportionate anger at such a trivial matter is a measure of how much importance Meg attached to her role of being the good wife. She said:

...I'm so *damn mad* – I could just *storm* out of here in the *car*

Capps and Ochs note how Meg uses the present tense of an obviously long past event. That is how real it still is in her mind. She says she wanted to leave, but couldn't. Now, being nine months pregnant doesn't usually mean one can't leave the house and drive a car to some other destination. Were she to do that, however, she wouldn't be the good little housewife, so she was trapped. She has to stay where she doesn't want to: home. In another sense, when a woman is pregnant, she is trapped. She's going to have to have that baby, and, under most circumstances, when it comes, she's going to be very tied down because of it.

It seems to me that the data presented by Capps and Ochs clearly show that Meg feels trapped by her housewife and mother roles, but displaces that entrapment on to other situations she doesn't want to be in. In all instances, however, she preserves her identity as society's model of the good wife. Clearly, their collection of data, tape-recorded, then examined thoroughly afterwards, is a model for therapy. Logistically, especially given managed health care restrictions, it would not be possible for most therapists to transcribe and analyse tapes of patient interviews. Ideally, a trained linguist should be on staffs of mental health centres and even psychiatrists' offices to analyse tapes for therapists. The efficacy of an objective linguistic analysis has certainly been shown by many books and articles, like those of Capps and Ochs, Beach,[40] Ferarra,[41] Mishler[42] and Chaika.[43] As Capps and Ochs say[44] 'We encourage psychotherapists to explore linguistic perspectives through cross-disciplinary collaboration and training. At the same time we encourage linguists to work with clinicians to develop more acute understandings of the interface of language and emotion.'

They lie

The word *lie* indicates an intentional distortion of the truth. The liar knows that he or she is not telling the truth, but intends the listener to think that the truth is being told. The question of why people would lie to their therapists came back to me time and again. Why would people pay good money to therapists and then lie to them? What kinds of lies did people create? People researching how people construct their lives through narrative have discovered that the narratives aren't always consistent, but there are reasons that stories change over time.

Linde[45] found that as people gain new experiences or change their minds about theories or gain new understandings, their life stories change. Anecdotes drop out of their repertoire, or are viewed from a different stance according to their new purposes. She reports on a young man who told her he had dropped out of science because of a horrible job he had in which he had to irradiate mice and 'then kill and dissect them in order to replicate some result that had already been established'. This inhumane task led him to reject science 'as a fundamentally inhumane and repulsive activity'. Linde met up with this man a few years later when he was planning to go on to graduate school in geology which was, in effect, a return to science. This time, in recounting his turnabout, he never mentioned the mousekilling episodes. Even when Linde reminded him that he had sworn off science after his last job, he just said, 'I dunno, just didn't like it. No accounting for taste, you know.' She could not elicit the mouse murders from him at all, despite the fact that they played such a vivid role in his earlier stories. I suspect that one explanation for this is that mouse killing plays no role in geology so that it wasn't brought to the fore. That is, geology does not readily lend itself to recalling mouse killings in a lab that used animals, since the labs he would now be experimenting in, so far as I have been able to determine, do not use animals.

Linde also tells the story of a young retarded man who spent a good deal of time trying to prove that retarded people may be far more able than others think. At some point, however, he decided he wasn't retarded after all, and the competencies and achievements that he earlier used to cite to prove that retarded people can be quite competent, he now used to prove that he wasn't and never had been retarded!

Are these lies? Or is it that life is not static for most people. It is entirely possible to reinterpret old events in light of new experiences and to come up with new understandings. If it weren't, we'd never be able to change our minds. Except for the Clives, Nates, Megs and Esthers among us, most of us do change our minds. And those who didn't change theirs because their self-narratives were frozen, being kept alive in their original state by repeated retellings, allowed no new points of view to be examined, no new interpretations, even healing ones.

Kathleen Ferrara[46] notes that therapists not only expect recurrences of narratives, but that 'Each retelling shows a different facet of the same thing.' It is from these different facets that clients and therapists both gain new insights. Ferrara claims that 'If storytelling in therapy becomes too ritualized, too pat, the therapist feels that progress is not being made.' Therapists should realize that ritualized retellings, such as those we have seen in this chapter, lead only to rigidity and resistance to change.

Capps and Ochs[47] point out that 'our memories are not snapshots of our experiences' and that 'we store our experiences in memory in connection with a web of associations'. Then, when we are retelling narratives, we may recall the memory in connection with associations different from those of a prior telling. Again, we may come up with a new interpretation. Ferrara[48] shows that retellings arise because the purpose of a narrative is to make a point and that point can change in different speech contexts. Narratives are a *flexible* (italics hers) resource.

Schafer,[49] speaking from the vantage of psychoanalysis puts it a bit differently. He points out that we change many aspects of our autobiographies as we change the implied or stated questions to which they are the answers. In addition, analysis changes the questions one addresses to the tale of one's life. Although he was talking of traditional psychoanalysis, the same may occur in any kind of therapy. When the therapist, psychoanalyst or not, interprets what the client says, the former is retelling the stories: certain features are related to others in new ways, or for the first time. One example is Capps and Ochs's retelling of Meg's life to show the connection between her not wanting to go somewhere, but going anyway, followed by the later panic attacks. As we have seen, they show that the panic attacks are not, as Meg perceives them, 'out of the blue'. A second example is my addition to Capps and Ochs's insights, showing the connection between people's need to behave in accordance with social norms and Meg's panic attacks. It was Capps and Ochs's retelling that led me to my conclusions. Had an analyst led Meg first to see that her attacks emanated from her own failure to refuse to go, then her life story might have been rewritten so that adverbs like 'out of the blue' wouldn't be used in her recounting of the panic attacks. Then, if a therapist had examined with Meg her conception of the duties of a wife and her actual feelings about those duties, together they might have interpreted as I did. Again, then, the panic attacks would take on new meanings. Indeed, one wonders in that case if Meg would have continued telling and retelling those stories as she did.

Many studies, such as those of Chafe,[50] Reason,[51] and Baars,[52] have shown that we cannot keep too much information in our focal memory at any one time. Memory is like vision in that respect. However, what is in focus, mentally or visually, does bring up associated memories which are then in a standby status and are accessed as we change our focal points. Given the enormous number of associations that any one word or memory can have, it is not surprising, then, that a memory accessed at different times carries with it different associations, and these associations may cast a new and different light on the memory.

Also, as this chapter has repeatedly shown, people always cast themselves in a moral light. If they perceive that a story they have told was received unfavourably by other interactors at another time, they may change the story to make it more morally fit, or may simply forget it. That is, like the mouse murderer mentioned above, they don't access it even when one might think it should be available to them.

In sum

Both therapist and client bring their entire linguistic repertoires into the therapeutic session. The therapist also has to encourage clients to speak by employing the noises, remarks and kinesics of ordinary interaction in the extraordinary interaction of therapy. Therapists have to learn to ask questions unconstrained by cultural bias, but acknowledging cultural realities. Therapists also have to consider each session as but a small chapter in the entire sequence of interviews, for then connections at first hidden will come to the fore. Therapists have to be especially sensitive to the fact that everybody's language system is a little bit different from everyone else's, that the meaning a therapist intends can, therefore, be misunderstood by a client, as well as the reverse. Words gain meaning by an individual's experience of them. The therapist has to be sensitive to sentence form as well. Does the client consistently or usually employ sentence transformations which avoid agents, especially 'I'? Does the client use adverbials indicating that things happen randomly or does the client use those that tie together events, showing cause and result? Does the client change his or her stories as he or she gains new understandings? Therapists must learn to value tropes: proverbs, idioms and metaphors. This doesn't mean that these should be used *ad nauseum*, but, where appropriate to enhance behaviour change, to build up rapport, to remove the directness of a painful subject, or to make the conclusions of the therapy session more vivid, hence memorable.

It is my position that effective therapy not only has to understand language and how it is used, but also, given the ephemeral nature of the spoken linguistic message, a record must be made of the interviews. To really analyse a client's narratives as well as the efficacy of the therapist's responses, interviews are best tape recorded and then listened to from time to time as therapy is progressing. I realize that most therapists literally don't have time to do a full-blown linguistic analysis of every session or even of one, but simply listening, in and of itself, will cause certain remarks or patterns to jump out at the therapist. Syntactic structures may be missed in the heat of face-to-face interaction. Revealing metaphors may have gone unnoticed at the time of their creation. The therapist might see questions that should have been raised but weren't. Connections might be found between events which, at first hearing, didn't seem connected at all. Patterns emerge at every level of language, linguistically and pragmatically. With the exception of Helena, the studies cited in this book were all tape-recorded, and Helena kept a diary which she filled in as soon as each session was over.

As noted at the outset of this book, the insights gathered by sociolinguistic investigation of how people use language are of great value to mental health therapists. The studies I cite from this field take language analysis far above the level of conjecture and empty theorizing. Rather, conclusions are drawn from replicable experiments and studies. These, along with the findings of cognitive linguistics, inform the analyses of behaviour presented in this volume.

Notes

1. Capps L, Ochs E (1995) Constructing Panic: The Discourse of Agoraphobia. Cambridge, Mass.: Harvard University Press,18.
2. Ibid., 175.
3. Bamberg M (1997) A constructivist approach to narrative development. In Bamberg E (ed) Narrative Development: Six Approaches. Mahwah, New Jersey: Lawrence Erlbaum Associates, 89.

4. Linde C (1993) Life Stories: The Creation of Coherence. New York: Oxford University Press, 101.

5. Capps and Ochs, Constructing Panic, 175.

6. Schafer R (1992) Retelling a Life. New York: Basic Books, Division of HarperCollins, xv.

7. In the UK, speech therapists actually deal with mentally ill patients and engage in psychotherapy with them. In the US, psychiatric social workers, certain trained registered nurses, and people with education degrees in counselling do this work, but speech therapists do not.

8. Pollio HR, Barlow JM, Fine HJ, Pollio MR (eds) (1977) Psychology and the Poetics of Growth: Figurative Language in Psychology, Psychotherapy, and Education. Hillsdale, NJ: Lawrence Erlbaum Publishers, 175.

9. Linde, Life Stories, 3.

10. Goffman E (1972) The moral career of the mental patient. In Manis J, Meltzer B (eds) Symbolic Interaction: A Reader in Social Psychology. Boston, Mass.: Allyn & Bacon, 542–3.

11. Goffman E (1955) On face work. Psychiatry 18: 213–31.

12. Abrahams RD (1972) The training of the man of words in talking sweet. Language in Society 1: 15-30; Chaika E (1994) Language: The Social Mirror, 3rd edn. Boston, Mass.: Heinle & Heinle, 214–28.

13. As was typical in the social sciences until the past decade or so, all pronouncements about speech behaviours were based upon male behaviours. Women were, by and large, not studied. We know women did not engage in the kinds of oral gaming males did, nor were they deacons at church, although women did hold other positions of authority there. The 'Amen Corner' was typically a female-dominated force in churches, but we know more about male African American preachers and male street poets than we do about female African American speakers.

14. In the United States today, Hispanics have maintained Spanish for the same purpose, and African Americans often retain Ebonics as a mode of bonding with each other and separating themselves from the society which has rejected them.

15. Chaika, Language, the Social Mirror, 3rd Ed, 217–28.

16. Ibid., 222–5.

17. Ibid., 81–118.

18. Labov W (1972) Rules for ritual insults. In Language in the Inner City. Philadelphia: University of Pennsylvania Press, 297–353.

19. Chaika, Language, the Social Mirror, 3rd Ed, 226–8.

20. Malinowski B (1923) Phatic communication. In Ogden CK, Richards IA (eds) The Meaning of Meaning (Supplement). London: Routledge & Kegan-Paul.

21. Milroy L (1980) Language and Social Networks. Baltimore: University Park Press.

22. Labov W (1966) The Social Stratification of English in New York City. Washington, DC: Center for Applied Linguistics.
23. Labov W, Robins C, Lewis J, Cohen P (1968) A Study of the English of Negro and Puerto Rican Speakers in New York City. Philadelphia: US Regional Survey.
24. This may not be true of all societies, however. Studies in Northern Ireland by Leslie Milroy (Milroy L (1980) Language and Social Networks. Baltimore: University Park Press) and in parts of England by Peter Trudgill (Trudgill P (1972) Sex, covert prestige, and linguistic change in the urban British English of Norwich. Language in Society 1: 179–95) indicate that in some places it is more important to speak like one's cohorts than to speak with educated social standards. The differences might have to do with general social mobility in different countries.
25. This does not mean that all newscasters in the United States speak the same way. They don't, but people perceive them as all speaking alike, and they consider this a 'neutral' way of speaking; hence, 'proper'. Educated people are speaking more and more alike in some respects, but there is much variation in vowel and intonation pronunciations both regionally and between older and younger speakers.
26. The same, of course, is true of females.
27. Labov, Social Stratification.
28. This is part of a Federal government programme in which the elderly are provided with one hot meal a day at various sites throughout each state.
29. *Home work* was factory work done at night at home and the worker was paid by the piece. In this instance, Esther made velvet jewellery boxes at night for a local jewellery firm.
30. Actually, although her aid was indispensable to her brothers, the truth is that they, too, worked hard both at outside jobs as well as at their school work so they were able to maximize their getting of scholar-ships and fellowships when these were available.
31. Actually, it has occurred to me that these two were an example of *folie à deux*. Although Al was unfailingly sweet and docile, he still believed every one of Esther's stories as she told them. He himself never repeated any, but he knew them by heart and assented to them all.
32. Leff J, Vaughn C (1985) Expressed Emotion in Families: Its Significance for Mental Illness. New York: The Guilford Press.
33. To be fair, it must be noted that Esther had lived through pogroms and had also often witnessed Jews being taunted and beaten by Ukrainian Christian townspeople. When she came to America, she was called 'Kike' and 'dirty Jew' and had seen her brothers being physically attacked because they were Jews.
34. Johnstone B (1996) The Linguistic Individual: Self-Expression in Language and Linguistics. New York: Oxford University Press.

35. Capps and Ochs, Panic, 57.
36. Ibid., 63.
37. Ibid., 108.
38. Ibid., 109.
39. Linde, Life Stories.
40. Beach WA (1996) Conversations about Illness: Family Preoccupations with Bulimia. Mahwah, New Jersey: Lawrence Erlbaum Associates.
41. Ferrara KW (1994) Therapeutic Ways with Words. New York: Oxford University Press.
42. Mishler EG (1984) The Discourse of Medicine: Dialectics of Medical Interviews. NJ: Ablex.
43. Chaika E (1981) How shall a discourse be understood? Discourse Processes 4: 71–87; Chaika E (1990) Understanding Psychotic Speech: Beyond Freud and Chomsky. Springfield, Illinois: Charles C Thomas.
44. Capps and Ochs, Panic, 174.
45. Linde, Life Stories, 32–3.
46. Ferrara, Therapeutic Words, 53.
47. Capps and Ochs, Panic, 15.
48. Ferrara, Therapeutic Words, 58.
49. Schafer R (1981) Narration in the psychoanalytic dialogue. In Mitchell WJT (ed) On Narrative. Chicago: University of Chicago Press, 31.
50. Chafe W (1994) Discourse, Consciousness, and Time. Chicago: University of Chicago Press.
51. Reason J (1984) Lapses of attention in everyday life. In Parasuraman R, Davies DR (eds) Varieties of Attention. New York: Academic Press.
52. Baars BJ (ed) (1992) Experimental Slips and Human Error: Exploring the Architecture of Volition. New York: Plenum Press.

Bibliography

Abrahams RD (1972) The training of the man of words in talking sweet. Language in Society 1: 15–30.

Abrahamson D (1997) Social networks and their development in the community. In France J, Muir N (eds) Communication and the Mentally Ill Patient: Developmental and Linguistic Approaches to Schizophrenia. London: Jessica Kingsley. pp 153–8.

Austin JL (1975) How to Do Things with Words, 2nd edn, Urmson JO, Sbisè M (eds). Cambridge, Mass.: Harvard University Press.

Baars BJ (ed) (1988) Cognitive Theory of Consciousness. Cambridge: Cambridge University.

Baars BJ (ed) (1992) Experimental Slips and Human Error: Exploring the Architecture of Volition. New York: Plenum Press.

Bamberg M (1997) A constructivist approach to narrative development. In Bamberg E (ed) Narrative Development: Six Approaches. Mahwah, New Jersey: Lawrence Erlbaum Associates. pp 89–132.

Bassin A (1984) Proverbs, slogans and folk sayings in the therapeutic community: a neglected therapeutic tool. Journal of Psychoactive Drugs 16: 51–6.

Bateson G (1972) Steps to an Ecology of Mind. New York: Ballantine.

Beach WA (1996) Conversations about Illness: Family Preoccupations with Bulimia. Mahwah, New Jersey: Lawrence Erlbaum Associates.

Beck B (1987) Metaphors, cognition, and artificial intelligence. In Haskell RE (1987) Cognition and Symbolic Structures: The Psychology of Metaphoric Transformation. Norwood, New Jersey: Ablex. pp 9–30.

Billow R et al. (1987) Metaphoric communication and miscommunication in schizophrenic and borderline states. In Haskell RE (ed) Cognition and Symbolic Structures: The Psychology of Metaphoric Transformation. Norwood, NJ: Ablex. pp 141–62.

Brown G, Yule G (1983) Discourse Analysis. New York: Cambridge University Press.

Brown J (1977) Mind, Brain, and Consciousness. New York: Academic Press.

Capps L, Ochs E (1995) Constructing Panic: The Discourse of Agoraphobia. Cambridge, Mass.: Harvard University Press.

Chafe W (1968) Idiomaticity as an anomaly in the Chomskyan paradigm. Foundations of Language 4: 109–27

Chafe W (1994) Discourse, Consciousness, and Time. Chicago: University of Chicago Press.

Chafe W (1998) Language and the flow of thought. In Tomasello M (ed) The New Psychology of Language: Cognitive and Functional Approaches to Language Structure. Mahwah: New Jersey: Lawrence Erlbaum Associates. pp 93–111.

Chaika E (1974) A linguist looks at 'schizophrenic' language. Brain and Language 1: 257–76.

Chaika E (1977) Schizophrenic speech, slips of the tongue, and jargonaphasia: a reply to Fromkin and to Lecours and Vaniers-Clement. Brain and Language 4: 464–75.

Chaika E (1981) How shall a discourse be understood? Discourse Processes 4: 71–87.

Chaika E (1982) A unified explanation for the diverse structural deviations reported for adult schizophrenics with disrupted speech. Journal of Communication Disorders 15: 167–89.

Chaika E (1982) Thought disorder or speech disorder in schizophrenia?' Schizophrenia Bulletin 8: 587–91.

Chaika E (1990) Understanding Psychotic Speech: Beyond Freud and Chomsky. Springfield, Illinois: Charles C Thomas.

Chaika E (1994) Language: The Social Mirror, 3rd edn. Boston, Mass.: Heinle & Heinle.

Chaika E (1995) On analysing schizophrenic speech: what model should we use?' In Sims A (ed) Speech and Language Disorders in Psychiatry. London: Gaskell. pp 47–56

Chaika E (1997) Intention, attention, and deviant schizophrenic speech. In France J, Muir N (eds) Communication and the Mentally Ill Patient. London: Jessica Kingsley Publishers. pp 18-29.

Chaika E, Alexander P (1986) The ice cream stories: a study in normal and psychotic narrations. Discourse Processes 9. pp 305–28.

Chaika E, Lambe R (1985) The locus of dysfunction of schizophrenic speech. Schizophrenia Bulletin 11: 8–14.

Chaika E, Lambe R (1986) Is schizophrenia a semiotic disorder? a reply to Lanin-Kettering and Harrow. Schizophrenia Bulletin 12.

Chapman J (1966) The early symptoms of schizophrenia. British Journal of Psychiatry 112: 225–51.

Chapman L, Chapman J, Daut R (1976) Schizophrenic inability to disattend from strong aspects of meaning. Journal of Abnormal Psychology 85: 35–40.

Chimombo M, Roseberry R (1998) The Power of Discourse: An Introduction to Discourse Analysis. Mahwah, New Jersey: Lawrence Erlbaum Associates.

Clark H, Lucy P (1975) Understanding what is meant from what is said: a study in conversationally conveyed requests. Journal of Verbal Learning and Verbal Behavior 14: 56–72.

Cohen B (1978) Referent communication disturbances in schizophrenia. In Schwartz S (ed) Language and Cognition in Schizophrenia. Hilldale, N.J.: Lawrence Erlbaum Publishers.

Crow TJ (1998) Nuclear symptoms as a window on the relationship between thought and speech. British Journal of Psychiatry 173: 303–9.

Crow TJ, Done J, Sacker A (1995) Childhood precursors of psychosis as clues to its evolutionary origins. European Archives of Psychiatry and Clinical Neuroscience 245: 61–9.

Dell G, Reich P (1977) To err is (no longer necessarily) human. Interfaces 6: 9–12.

Diver W (1977) A concise grammar of English grammar I. In Diver W (ed) Columbia University Working Papers in Linguistics. New York: Columbia University. pp 1–20.

Docherty N, DeRosa M, Andreasen NC (1996) Communication disturbances in schizophrenia and mania. Archives of General Psychiatry 53: 358–64.

Duffley PJ (1992) The English Infinitive. English Language Series. New York: Longman.

Erickson F (1984) Rhetoric, anecdote, and rhapsody: coherence strategies in a conversation among Black American adolescents. In Tannen D (ed) Coherence in Spoken and Written Discourse, Norwood, NJ: Ablex. pp 81–154.

Erickson F, Shultz J (1982) The Counselor as Gatekeeper: Social Interaction in Interviews. New York: Academic Press.

Fairclough N (1989) Language and Power. Language in Social Life Series. New York: Longman.

Ferrara KW (1994a) Repetition as rejoinder in therapeutic discourse: echoing and mirroring. In Johnstone B (ed) Repetition in Discourse: Interdisciplinary Perspectives, Vol. 2, Advances in Discourse Processes. Norwood, NJ: Ablex. pp 66–83.

Ferrara KW (1994b) Therapeutic Ways with Words. New York: Oxford University Press.

Fillmore CJ (1968) The case for case. In Bach E, Harms E (eds) Universals in Linguistic Theory. New York: Holt, Rinehart & Winston. pp 1–90.

Forrest D (1976) Nonsense and sense in schizophrenic language. Schizophrenia Bulletin 2: 286–98.

Francis WN (1954) The Structure of American English. New York: Ronald Press.

Freyer F (1997) There's more to it than 'talk'. The Providence Sunday Journal, 26 October 1997, L2.

Frith C (1997) Language and communication in schizophrenia. In Communication and the Mentally Ill Patient. London: Jessica Kingsley. pp 10–17.

Fromkin V (1975) A linguist looks at 'A linguist looks at "schizophrenic" language'. Brain and Language 2: 498–503.

Gazzaniga M (1992) Nature's Mind: The Biological Roots of Thinking, Emotions, Sexuality, Language, and Intelligence. New York: Basic Books.

Gibbs RW Jr (1987) What does it mean to say that a metaphor has been understood? In Haskell RE (ed) Cognition and Symbolic Structures: The Psychology of Metaphoric Transformation. Norwood, NJ: Ablex. pp 31–48.

Giles H, Taylor D, Bourhis R (1973) Towards a theory of interpersonal accommodations through language: some Canadian data. Language in Society 2: 177–223

Gilligan C (1982) In a Different Voice: Women's Conception of Self and Morality. Cambridge, Mass.: Harvard University Press.

Goffman E (1955) On face work. Psychiatry 18: 213–31.

Goffman E (1968) Asylums: Essays on the Social Situations of Mental Patients and Other Inmates. London: Penguin Books.

Goffman E (1972) The moral career of the mental patient. In Manis J, Meltzer B (eds) Symbolic Interaction: A Reader in Social Psychology. Boston, Mass.: Allyn & Bacon. pp 234–44.

Goffman E (1974) Frame Analysis: An Essay on the Organization of Experience. Cambridge, Mass: Harvard University Press.

Goffman E (1981) Forms of Talk. Philadelphia: University of Pennsylvania Press.

Haiman J (1998) Talk is Cheap: Sarcasm, Alienation, and the Evolution of Language. New York: Oxford University Press.

Halliday MAK (1985) An Introduction to Functional Grammar. Baltimore: Edward Arnold.

Hallowell EM, Smith HF (1983) Communication through poetry in the therapy of a schizophrenic patient. Journal of the American Academy of Psychoanalysis 11: 133–58.

Hanks WF (1996) Language and Communicative Practices. Boulder, Colorado: Westview Press.

Hayes C (1997) Applying personal construct psychology. In France J, Muir N (eds)

Communication and the Mentally Ill Patient: Developmental and Linguistic Approaches to Schizophrenia. London: Jessica Kingsley. pp 127–38.

Heine B (1997) Cognitive Foundations of Grammar. New York: Oxford University Press.

Heine B, Claudi U, Hünnemeyer F (1991) Grammaticalization: A Conceptual Framework. Chicago: University of Chicago Press.

Herbert R, Waltensperger K (1980) Schizophrasia: a case study of a paranoid schizophrenic's language. Applied Psycholinguistics 1: 81–93.

Herbert RK, Waltensperger KZ (1982) Linguistics, psychology, and psychopathology: the case of schizophrenic language. In Obler L, Menne L (eds) Exceptional Language and Linguistics. New York: Academic Press.

Hodel B, Brenner M, Merlo G, Teuber F (1998) Emotional management therapy in early psychosis. British Journal of Psychiatry 173: 126–33.

Honeck RP (1997) A Proverb in Mind: The Cognitive Science of Proverbial Wit and Wisdom. Mahwah, New Jersey: Lawrence Erlbaum Associates.

Jack D (1991) Silencing the Self. Cambridge, Mass.: Harvard University Press.

Johnstone B (1996) The Linguistic Individual: Self-Expression in Language and Linguistics. New York: Oxford University Press.

Kay P, Kempton E (1984) What is the Sapir–Whorf Hypothesis? American Anthropologist 86: 65–79.

Kean ML (1980) Grammatical representations and the description of language processing. In Caplan D (ed) Biological Studies of Mental Processes. Cambridge, Mass: MIT Press.

Kuno S (1987) Functional Syntax: Anaphora, Discourse, and Empathy. Chicago: University of Chicago Press.

Labov W (1963) The social motivation of a sound change. Word 19: 273–309.

Labov W (1966) The Social Stratification of English in New York City. Washington, DC: Center for Applied Linguistics.

Labov W (1972) Rules for ritual insults. In Language in the Inner City. Philadelphia: University of Pennsylvania Press. pp 297–353.

Labov W, Fanshel D (1977) Therapeutic Discourse. New York: Academic Press.

Labov W, Robins C, Lewis J, Cohen P (1968) A Study of the English of Negro and Puerto Rican Speakers in New York City. Philadelphia: US Regional Survey.

Laffal J (1965) Pathological and Normal Language. New York: Atherton Press.

Laing RD (1967) The Politics of Experience and The Bird of Paradise. Harmondsworth, Middlesex: Penguin.

Lakoff G (1987) Women, Fire, and Dangerous Things: What Categories Reveal about the Mind. Chicago: University of Chicago Press, 1987).

Lakoff G, Johnson M (1980) Metaphors We Live By. Chicago: University of Chicago Press.

Lakoff G, Turner M (1989) More Than Cool Reason: A Field Guide to Poetic Metaphor. Chicago: University of Chicago Press.

Lakoff R (1972) Language in context. Language 48: 907–27.

Langacker R (1998) Conceptualization, symbolization,and grammar. In Tomasello M (ed) The New Psychology of Language: Cognitive and Functional Approaches to Language Structure. Mahwah: New Jersey: Lawrence Erlbaum Associates. pp 1–39

Leff J, Vaughn C (1985) Expressed Emotion in Families: Its Significance for Mental Illness. New York: The Guilford Press.

Lehrer A (1983) The Semantics of Wine Tasting. Bloomington: Indiana University Press.

Levin B (1993) English Verb Classes and Alternations. Chicago: University of Chicago Press.

Levin SR (1977) The Semantics of Metaphor. Baltimore: Johns Hopkins University Press.

Linde C (1993) Life Stories: The Creation of Coherence. New York: Oxford University Press.

Lorenz M (1961) Problems posed by schizophrenic language. Archives of General Psychiatry 4: 603–10.

Macdonald L (1997) Neuro Linguistic Programming as an experiential constructivist therapy for semantic pragmatic disorder. In France J, Muir N (eds) Communication and the Mentally Ill Patient: Developmental and Linguistic Approaches to Schizophrenia. London: Jessica Kingsley, 139–52.

Macedo D (1994) Literacies of Power: What Americans Are Not Allowed to Know. Boulder: Westview Press.

Maher B (1972) The language of schizophrenia: a review and an interpretation. British Journal of Psychiatry 120: 4–17.

Maher B (1968) The shattered language of schizophrenia. Psychiatry Today, November.

Malinowski B (1923) Phatic communication. In Ogden CK, Richards IA (eds) The Meaning of Meaning (Supplement). London: Routledge & Kegan-Paul.

McCawley J (1968) Lexical insertion in a transformational grammar without deep structure. Papers from the Fourth Regional Meeting of the Chicago Linguistic Society: 71–80.

Miller GA (1982) Some problems in the theory of demonstrative reference. In Jarvella R, Klein W (eds) Speech, Place, and Action. New York: John Wiley. pp 61–72.

Miller J (1995) Does spoken language have sentences? In Palmer FR (ed) Grammar and Meaning: Essays in Honour of Sir John Lyons. New York: Cambridge University Press. pp 116–35.

Milroy L (1980) Language and Social Networks. Baltimore: University Park Press.

Mishler EG (1984) The Discourse of Medicine: Dialectics of Medical Interviews. NJ: Ablex.

Morice R (1995) Language impairments and executive dysfunction in schizophrenia. In Sims A (ed) Speech and Language Disorders in Psychiatry. London: Gaskell. pp 57–69.

Morice RD, Ingram JC (1982) Language analysis in schizophrenia: diagnostic implications. Australian and New Zealand Journal of Psychiatry 16: 11–21.

Muir N (1997) Semantic pragmatic disorder and the role of the speech and language therapist in psychiatry. In France J, Muir N (eds) Communication and the Mentally Ill Patient: Developmental and Linguistic Approaches to Schizophrenia. London: Jessica Kingsley. pp 117–26.

Noel-Jorand MC, Reinert M, Giudicelli S, Dassa D (1997) A new approach to discourse analysis in psychiatry, applied to a schizophrenic patient's speech. Schizophrenia Research 25: 186–97.

Philips SU (1970) Acquisition of rules for appropriate speech usage. In Alatis J (ed) Bilingualism and Language: Anthropological, Linguistic, Psychological, and Sociological Aspects, Monograph series on Languages and Linguistics.Washington, DC: Georgetown University Press.

Philips SU (1976) Some sources of cultural variability in the regulation of talk. Language in Society 5: 81–95.

Pollio HR, Barlow JM, Fine HJ, Pollio MR (eds) (1977) Psychology and the Poetics of Growth: Figurative Language in Psychology, Psychotherapy, and Education. Hillsdale, NJ: Lawrence Erlbaum Publishers.

Quirk R, Greenbaum S (1973) A Concise Grammar of Contemporary English. New York: Harcourt Brace Jovanovich.

Quirk R, Svartvik J (1966) Investigating Linguistic Acceptability, The Hague: Mouton.

Radford A (1981) Transformational Syntax: A Student's Guide to Chomsky's Extended Standard Theory. New York: Cambridge University Press.

Reason J (1984) Lapses of attention in everyday life. In Parasuraman R, Davies DR (eds) Varieties of Attention. New York: Academic Press.

Ribeiro BT (1994) Coherence in Psychotic Discourse. New York: Oxford University Press.

Rochester S, Martin J (1979) Crazy Talk: A Study of the Discourse of Schizophrenic Speakers, New York: Plenum Press.

Rogers TB (1989) The use of slogans, colloquialisms, and proverbs in the treatment of substance addiction: a psychological application of proverbs. Proverbium 6: 103–12.

Rumelhart D (1979) Some problems with the notion of literal meanings. In Ortony A (ed) Metaphor and Thought. New York: Cambridge University Press. pp 78–90.

Sacks H (1972) An initial investigation of the usability of conversational data for doing sociology. In Sudnow D (ed) Studies in Social Interaction. New York: Free Press.

Sacks H (1992) Lectures on Conversation, Vol. 1, Jefferson G (ed). Cambridge, Mass.: Blackwell.

Schafer R (1981) Narration in the psychoanalytic dialogue. In Mitchell WJT (ed) On Narrative. Chicago: University of Chicago Press. pp 25–49.

Schafer R (1992) Retelling a Life. New York: Basic Books, Division of HarperCollins.

Searle JR (1969) Speech Acts: An Essay in the Philosophy of Language. Cambridge: Cambridge University Press.

Sells P (1985) Lectures on Contemporary Syntactic Theories: An Introduction to Government-Binding Theory, Generalized Phrase Structure Grammar, and Lexical-Functional Grammar. Stanford, CA: CSLI/Stanford.

Sternberg R, Tourangeau R, Nigro G (1979) Metaphor, induction, and social policy: the convergence of macroscopic and microscopic views. In Ortony A (ed) Metaphor and Thought. New York: Cambridge University Press. pp 325–53.

Sullivan C (1986) The therapeutic functions of metaphor. Journal of Communication Therapy 4: 138–46.

Svartvik J (1966) On Voice in the English Verb. The Hague: Mouton

Szasz TS (1973) The Age of Madness: The History of Involuntary Mental Hospitalization Presented in Selected Texts. Garden City, New York: Doubleday, Anchor.

Tannen D (1984) Conversational Style. Norwood, N.J.: Ablex.

Thomas P (1994) A Manual for the Brief Syntactic Analysis, mimeo.

Thomas P, Leudar I (1995) Syntactic processing and communication disorder in first-onset schizophrenia. In Sims A (ed) Speech and Language Disorders in Psychiatry. London: Gaskell. pp 96–112.

Trudgill P (1972) Sex, covert prestige, and linguistic change in the urban British English of Norwich. Language in Society 1: 179–95.

Turner M (1996) The Literary Mind: The Origins of Thought and Language. New York: Oxford University Press.

Turner V (1974) Dramas, Fields, and Metaphors. Ithaca, New York: Cornell University Press.

van Dijk T (1988) News as Discourse. Hillsdale, NJ: Lawrence Erlbaum.

Vetter H (1968) Language Behavior in Schizophrenia. Springfield, Ill: Charles C Thomas.

Walsh I (1997) Conversational skills and schizophrenia: an exploration. In France J, Muir N (eds) Communication and the Mentally Ill Patient. London: Jessica Kingsley. 98–116.

Whaley BB (1993) When 'try, try again' turns to 'you're beating a dead horse': the rhetorical characteristics of proverbs and their potential for influencing therapeutic change. Metaphor and Symbolic Activity 8: 127–39.

White H (1981) The value of narrativity in the representation of reality. In Mitchell WJT (ed) On Narrative. Chicago: University of Chicago Press. pp 1–23.

Index